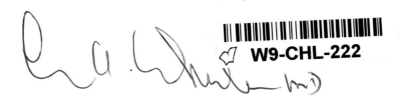

Guide
for Adult
Immunization

Third Edition

Printing and distribution of this copy of *Guide for Adult Immunization* was supported by grants from: SmithKline Beecham Pharmaceuticals, Connaught Laboratories, Lederle-Praxis Biologicals, and Merck & Company. The development and content of the *Guide* was directed entirely by representatives of the American College of Physicians and the Infectious Diseases Society of America.

Guide
for Adult
Immunization

Third Edition

ACP Task Force on Adult Immunization
and
Infectious Diseases Society of America

Published by the American College of Physicians
Philadelphia, Pennsylvania

Also Available from the American College of Physicians

American College of Physicians Home Care Guide: Cancer
Clinical Practice Guidelines
Common Diagnostic Tests: Use and Interpretation - Second Edition
Common Screening Tests
Diagnostic Strategies for Common Medical Problems
Drug Prescribing in Renal Failure - Third Edition
Software for Internists

Publications from the *British Medical Journal* are now distributed in North America by the American College of Physicians

Publications catalogue and ordering information for American College of Physicians and *British Medical Journal* publications are available from:

Customer Service
American College of Physicians
Independence Mall West
Sixth Street at Race
Philadelphia, PA 19106-1572
(215) 351-2600
(800) 523-1546

Second Edition

Printed in the United States of America

Library of Congress Cataloging-in-Publication Data
Main entry under title:

Guide for adult immunization/ACP Task Force on Adult Immunization and Infectious Diseases Society of America. - 3rd ed.
    p. cm.
    Includes bibliographical references and index.
    ISBN 0-943126-23-1
    1. Immunization—Handbooks, manuals, etc. 2. Vaccines
Handbooks, manuals, etc. 3. Immunization—United States—
Handbooks, manuals, etc. I. American College of Physicians. Task
Force on Adult Immunization. II. Infectious Diseases Society of
America. [DNLM: 1. Immunization—handbooks. 2. Vaccines—
handbooks. 3. Communicable Disease Control—handbooks.
    QW 39 G946 1994]
RA638.G85   1994
614.4'7—dc20

Library of Congress Catalog Card No. 94-3075
ISBN 0-943126-23-1

Task Force on Adult Immunization

American College of Physicians

Pierce Gardner, MD, FACP, Task Force Chair, Professor of Medicine and Associate Dean for Academic Affairs, State University of New York, Stony Brook, NY

Marie Griffin, MD, MPH, FACP, Associate Professor, Departments of Preventive Medicine and Medicine, Vanderbilt University School of Medicine, Nashville, TN

Peter Gross, MD, FACP, Chairman, Department of Internal Medicine, Hackensack Medical Center, Hackensack, NJ, Professor of Medicine, New Jersey Medical School

F. Marc LaForce, MD, FACP, Physician-in-Chief, The Genesee Hospital, and Professor of Medicine, the University of Rochester School of Medicine and Dentistry, Rochester, NY

Infectious Diseases Society of America

William Schaffner, MD, FACP, Professor and Chairman, Department of Preventive Medicine, Professor of Medicine, Division of Infectious Diseases, Vanderbilt University School of Medicine, Nashville, TN

Theodore Eickhoff, MD, FACP, Professor of Medicine, Division of Infectious Disease, University of Colorado Health Sciences Center, Denver, CO

Centers for Disease Control and Prevention

Raymond Strikas, MD, FACP, National Immunization Program, Centers for Disease Control and Prevention, Atlanta, GA

Acknowledgments

The Task Force on Adult Immunization thanks the experts in the field who reviewed the manuscript or portions of it during the preparation of this Guide and provided valuable assistance and comments. We appreciate their advice and many useful suggestions.

We thank several staff members of the American College of Physicians who provided excellent ideas and exhibited diligence and patience in nurturing this publication: Linda Johnson White, Director, Department of Scientific Policy; Bobbie Lewis; and Ellen Marshall.

Pierce Gardner, MD, FACP, Chair
Theodore Eickhoff, MD, FACP
Marie Griffin, MD, MPH, FACP
Peter Gross, MD, FACP
F. Marc LaForce, MD, FACP
William Schaffner, MD, FACP
Raymond Strikas, MD, FACP

Contents

Introduction

The success of pediatric immunization programs has reduced the overall burden of preventable infections in children to new lows both in the United States and worldwide. However, immunization of adults does not receive the same priority as immunization of children, despite the fact that deaths from vaccine-preventable diseases occur predominantly in adults. In the United States, 50 000 to 70 000 estimated yearly deaths among adults from pneumococcal infection, influenza, and hepatitis B (Table 0.1) dwarf the annual mortality from diseases targeted by childhood immunizations (fewer than 500 deaths). Annual deaths from infections preventable by adult immunizations exceed those resulting from automobile accidents or the acquired immunodeficiency syndrome.

Factors contributing to this poor record include lingering doubts of both the public and health care providers about the efficacy and safety of vaccines; uncertainty regarding specific recommendations; concern about liability; inadequate reimbursement; and poorly developed systems for immunization of adults. Among the 19 vaccines provided for adults, insufficient attention is given to setting priorities that emphasize the vaccines that have the greatest potential effect on public health: pneumococcal vaccine, influenza vaccine, and hepatitis B vaccine. Notable preventive medicine successes in recent years have included marked reductions in deaths from cardiovascular disease, lung cancer, and automobile accidents. In each area, the public, the government, and the medical community have collaborated successfully. Adult death from vaccine-preventable disease is a problem of comparable magnitude and deserves a similar priority and collaborative effort.

New Recommendations

In writing the third edition of the *Guide for Adult Immunization,* the American College of Physicians Task Force on Adult Immunization tried to supplement the specific recommendations relating to the individual vaccines by addressing broader issues. A chapter on implementation strategies

TABLE 0.1. Estimates of the Effect of Full Use of the Vaccines Now Advocated for Adults

Diseases	Estimated Annual Deaths Among Adults	Estimated Vaccine Efficacy*	Current Vaccine Use[†]	Additional Preventable Deaths/Years[‡]
	n	%	%	*n*
Influenza	20 000[§]	70	30	9800
Pneumococcal infection	40 000	60	14	20 640
Hepatitis B	5000	90	10[‖]	4050
Tetanus/diphtheria	<25	99	40[¶]	<15
Traveler's diseases (Cholera, typhoid, Japanese encephalitis, yellow fever, poliomyelitis, rabies)	<10	—	—	<10
Measles, mumps, and rubella	<30	95	Varying	<30

* These composite estimates indicate efficacy in immunocompetent adults. In the elderly and immunocompromised, efficacy estimates are lower.
[†] Percentage of targeted groups that are in compliance with current recommendations. Rates vary among different targeted groups.
[‡] (Potential additional vaccine use) × (estimated vaccine efficacy) × (estimated annual deaths).
[§] Varying (range, 0 to 40 000).
[‖] Varies widely (1% to 60%) among different target groups.
[¶] Estimate based on seroprevalence data.
Source: Gardner P, Schaffner W. Immunization of adults. N Engl J Med. 1993;328:1252–8.

was added, and throughout the book attempts were made to set public health priorities for the measures considered. The Task Force also re-examined a number of well-established recommendations by critically reviewing the epidemiologic and immunologic evidence. This led to several new recommendations. Chief among these are:

- That age 50 years be established as a time for review of preventive health measures, with special emphasis on evaluating risk factors that would indicate a need for giving pneumococcal vaccine and initiating annual influenza immunization. Almost one third of Americans ages 50 to 64 years have risk factors for invasive pneumococcal disease, yet fewer than 10% have received the vaccine.

- That individuals who receive pneumococcal vaccine before age 65 years, because of their risk factors, should be considered candidates for reimmunization at age 65 years provided at least 6 years have passed since they received the first dose of pneumococcal vaccine.

- That as an equivalent alternative strategy to the current recommendation for routine tetanus and diphtheria (Td) boosters every 10 years, special emphasis be given to assure that all adults have completed a primary immunization series with tetanus and diphtheria toxoids, followed by a single mid-life Td booster at age 50 years for individuals who have completed the full pediatric series, including the teenage/young adult booster. The recommendation for Td boosters as part of wound management is unchanged.

- That the use of amantadine/rimantadine prophylaxis for influenza A be more cautious, recognizing the concern that many physicians have expressed regarding adverse neurologic reactions to amantadine in their elderly patients. It is anticipated that rimantadine will be better tolerated.

- That the serologic response to hepatitis B immunization be assessed in all vaccine recipients older than 30 years, recognizing that seroconversion rates diminish with age.

The new recommendations are explained in detail in subsequent chapters.

How the *Guide* Is Arranged

As in previous editions, the immunization needs of various groups of patients are identified, and essential information on the effectiveness, clinical indications, administration, adverse effects, precautions, and contraindications for all licensed vaccines and immune globulin preparations is provided. The *Guide* is deliberately repetitious; it is organized by type of patient and by specific vaccines or immune globulins to increase its convenience as a ready reference for busy practitioners.

In most instances, information needed to treat individual patients can be found in one section of Chapters 2 to 7. Specific details on the use of individual vaccines or immune globulins are discussed in Chapter 8. In addition, the tables and appendices provide immediate access to clinically useful information. Tables 0.2 and 0.3 in this introduction summarize the universal childhood and adult vaccine recommendations by age. Appendix 1 presents the immunization schedules, indications, precautions and contraindications, and other special considerations for each licensed immunobiologic agent. Appendix 2 lists available immunobiologic agents according to product name and manufacturer. Appendix 3 provides a complete reference to the most recent recommendations of the Advisory Committee on Immunization Practices published in *Morbidity and Mortality Weekly Report*. Appendix 4 outlines state immunization requirements for schools and colleges, Appendix 5 provides the addresses and telephone numbers for each state and territorial health department, and Appendix 6 lists other sources

TABLE 0.2. Recommended Schedule for Routine Active Immunization of Healthy Infants and Children*

Vaccine	At Birth (before hospital discharge)	1–2	2†	4	6	6–18	12–15	4–6 (before school entry)
		←———————— months ————————→						years
DTP	—	—	DTP	DTP	DTP	—	DTP(DTaP)‡	DTaP (DTP)
OPV	—	—	OPV	OPV	OPV§	—	—	OPV
MMR	—	—	—	—	—	—	MMR	MMR‖
Hib¶								
A	—	—	Hib	Hib	Hib	—	Hib**	—
B	—	—	Hib	Hib	—	—	Hib**	—
HB††								
Option 1	HB	HB‡‡	—	—	—	HB‡‡	—	—
Option 2	—	HB‡‡	—	HB‡‡	—	HB‡‡	—	—

*DTP = Diphtheria, tetanus, and pertussis vaccine. A combined DTP and Hib vaccine is also available.

DTaP = Diphtheria, tetanus, and acellular pertussis vaccine. DTaP preparations are licensed only for use as the fourth and/or fifth doses of the DTP series among children ages 15 months through 6 years (before the seventh birthday).

OPV = Live oral polio vaccine.

MMR = Measles, mumps, and rubella vaccine.

Hib = *Haemophilus influenzae* type b conjugate vaccine. A combined DTP and Hib vaccine is also available. Recommended schedules vary by manufacturer. For recommendations specific to the vaccine being used, consult the package insert.

HB = Hepatitis B vaccine.

† Can begin at age 6 weeks.

‡ A minimum interval of 6 months is recommended between the third and fourth dose. DTaP preparations are currently licensed only for use as the fourth and/or fifth doses of the DTP series among children ages 15 months through 6 years (before the seventh birthday). Some experts prefer to give these vaccines at 18 months.

§ The American Academy of Pediatrics recommends this dose of vaccine at ages 6 to 18 months.

‖ The American Academy of Pediatrics recommends this dose of MMR vaccine be given at entry to middle school or junior high school.

¶ Schedule A: HbOC (Lederle Praxis) or PRP-T (Pasteur Merieux, distributed by SmithKline Beecham, and Connaught) or DTP-HbOC (Lederle Praxis)
Schedule B: PRP-OMP (Merck, Sharp & Dohme)

** After the primary infant Hib conjugate vaccine series is completed, any licensed Hib conjugate vaccine may be used as a booster dose at ages 12 to 15 months.

†† For infants born of hepatitis B surface antigen (HBsAg)-negative mothers. Premature infants of HBsAg-negative mothers should receive the first dose of the hepatitis B vaccine series at the time of hospital discharge or when the other routine childhood vaccines are initiated. (All infants born of HBsAg-positive mothers should receive immunoprophylaxis for hepatitis B as soon as possible after birth.)

‡‡ Hepatitis B vaccine can be given simultaneously with DTP (or DTaP), OPV, MMR, and/or Hib at the same visit.

TABLE 0.3.   Recommended Immunization Schedule for Adults

Age	Recommended Schedule
Teenagers/ Young Adults	Completion of all childhood primary immunizations Hepatitis B for those not immunized in childhood Td booster*
50 years	Completion of all primary immunizations[†] Td booster* Assessment of risk factors indicating need for pneumococcal vaccine and annual influenza immunization
65 years or older	Completion of all primary immunizations[†] Yearly influenza vaccine Pneumococcal vaccine[‡]

*Td = Tetanus and diptheria toxoids. The Task Force Adult Immunization endorses two strategies as equivalent: 1) the traditional recommendation of Td boosters every 10 years throughout life; and 2) special emphasis on completion of the primary immunization series followed by a single mid-life booster at age 50 years for individuals who have completed the full pediatric series including the teenage/young adult booster.

[†] Mainly Td. Individuals born before 1957 are not targeted for primary immunization for measles, mumps, or rubella. Similarly, poliomyelitis has become such a rare disease that primary immunization of older adults is not cost-effective.

[‡] Individuals who first receive pneumococcal vaccine 6 or more years before this age should be considered for reimmunization at age 65 years, although data are incomplete.

of vaccine information. Appendix 7 provides a model form for recording immunizations that can be included in patients' medical records. Appendix 8 presents an immunization record suitable for patient use. Because the National Childhood Vaccine Injury Act of 1986 requires that physicians and other health care providers report certain adverse reactions after the administration of selected vaccines, details regarding these reportable events and how they are to be reported are summarized in Appendices 9 and 10. Although the *Guide* is intended to provide the basic information necessary for patient immunization, in some instances more detailed information may be required. Appendix 11 contains selected references to supplement the guidelines.

History of the *Guide*

The first edition of the *Guide for Adult Immunization* was prepared by the Committee on Immunization of the Council of Medical Societies of the American College of Physicians in 1985. In 1987, the Committee was reorganized as the Task Force on Adult Immunization. At the same time, the College recognized that its concern for adult immunization was shared by the Infectious Diseases Society of America, and the Society was invited to join the College in supporting the Task Force and in preparing and sponsoring the second edition. This joint effort signified the renewed and expanded commitment of both organizations to foster a broader awareness of the benefits of adult immunization for patients and society at large. The third edition of the *Guide for Adult Immunization* continues that tradition and should provide physicians and other health care providers with the information they need to translate knowledge about immunization into effective clinical practice.

Every attempt was made to ensure the accuracy of the information contained in this *Guide;* however, physicians should refer to package inserts regarding correct dosages and recommended routes of administration for each vaccine. In addition, current information on the indications, contraindications, and adverse effects of vaccines, toxoids, and immune globulins is reported regularly in the *Morbidity and Mortality Weekly Report.* Readers are asked to contact the American College of Physicians immediately if any errors are found in the *Guide.*

1.

General Recommendations for Adult Immunization

Despite their success, childhood vaccination programs alone will not eliminate vaccine-preventable diseases. Many of these diseases occur among adolescents and adults, particularly those who have missed both natural infection and past immunization. Because some conditions are more serious (for example, measles) or may have devastating secondary consequences (for example, congenital rubella) when they occur in adults, physicians must ensure that their adult patients are protected. Fifty percent of the State legislatures have made prematriculation immunization mandatory for students of colleges and other post-secondary institutions (Appendix 4). The Occupational Safety and Health Administration requires certain employers to offer their employees hepatitis B vaccine. Other institutions also require that their students or employees be immunized against certain diseases.

A careful history of immunizations should be obtained from each new patient and reviewed periodically. This process should become as routine in the practice of physicians who treat adults as it is among pediatricians. The five vaccines listed in Table 1.1 are those used most often for routine adult immunization. Their schedules for use are summarized in Appendix 1. More details are provided in Chapter 8, which addresses each vaccine separately.

A patient's immunization history is determined most reliably by obtaining the information from records kept by the patient or by the patient's previous physician. Unfortunately, most adults do not have their own immunization records, and they may have received immunizations from several different providers in the past. Consequently, an accurate history is often difficult to obtain. As a rule, if there is doubt about previous immunizations, it is best to assume that patients are not immunized.

Age, military service, and occupation may help determine immunization history. Most persons born before 1957 can be considered immune to measles and mumps through natural infection. Persons who were 10 years or older when measles, mumps, and rubella vaccines were licensed (1963, 1967, and 1969, respectively) are less likely to have received these vaccines than are persons who were younger or who were born since then.

TABLE 1.1. Routine Immunization of Adults

Vaccine	Recommendations
Pneumococcal	All adults age ≥65 years; all younger adults with risk factors. Reimmunization is recommended at age 65 if 6 or more years have passed since first pneumococcal immunization
Influenza	Yearly for all adults age ≥65 years; all younger adults with risk factors. Offer to other healthy younger adults
Hepatitis B	Sexually active young adults; high-risk groups. Assess serologic response in persons age ≥30 years
Measles-mumps-rubella (MMR)	Adults born after 1956 without proof of immunity or documentation of previous immunization; two doses for special risk groups
Tetanus-diphtheria (Td)	Completion of primary (three-dose) immunization schedule followed by either Td boosters every 10 years, or a single mid-life (at age 50 years) booster for persons who have completed the full pediatric series, including the teenage/young adult booster

Consequently, the date of licensure for each vaccine provides useful information. All states require that children entering or attending school be immunized against certain infectious diseases (Appendix 4). However, variations exist in state laws and in their enforcement. Consequently, the fact that a young adult has recently been a high school student does not guarantee previous immunization. Persons with military experience are routinely immunized against diphtheria, tetanus, measles, rubella, and poliomyelitis, and some may receive special vaccines against diseases such as typhoid or Japanese encephalitis. Persons involved in specific occupations may already have received certain vaccines; for example, many veterinary students are routinely given pre-exposure rabies vaccine. Others who have traveled abroad may have received several vaccines (for example, typhoid and yellow fever vaccines). For some diseases (rubella and hepatitis B, for example), serologic testing can provide definitive information about immunity.

Contraindications to Immunization

Severe hypersensitivity reactions, including anaphylaxis after immunization, are rare. These reactions are almost always caused by hypersensitivity to one or more vaccine components (residual animal proteins, antibiotics, preservatives, or stabilizers). The most common allergic component is egg protein found in vaccines prepared in embryonated chicken eggs or chicken embryonal cultures (in measles, mumps, influenza, and yellow fever vaccines). Persons who eat eggs or egg-containing products can receive these vaccines. In general, persons with a history of anaphylactic reactions to eggs or egg proteins should not be vaccinated. However, if the physician decides the vaccine benefit outweighs the risk, protocols have been developed that enable such persons to be immunized (Appendix 11, Measles, reference 20).

On rare occasions, patients will have anaphylactic hypersensitivity to trace amounts of neomycin and streptomycin present in vaccines (for example, neomycin in measles, mumps, and rubella [MMR] vaccine). Vaccination may be contraindicated in such individuals. None of the currently licensed vaccines contains penicillin or any of its derivatives; consequently, a history of penicillin allergy is not a contraindication to vaccination. Sometimes, severe systemic reactions follow administration of cholera, typhoid, or plague vaccines. These reactions are poorly understood, but most probably represent toxic rather than true hypersensitivity reactions. Revaccination of such individuals should be avoided.

Immunizations with live virus vaccines should be avoided in patients who are immunocompromised as a result of disease or medical treatment or those who live in a household with such a person. Although the MMR vaccine (or its components) has been safely given to children infected with the human immunodeficiency virus (HIV), there is little information regarding the safety of these vaccines in HIV-infected adults. The Task Force on Adult Immunization recommends that asymptomatic HIV-infected individuals should receive MMR vaccine (or its components) when indicated, but for individuals who have progressed to the acquired immunodeficiency syndrome (AIDS), the decision should be based on the degree of immunosuppression and the likelihood of exposure to measles, mumps, or rubella. Persons with leukemia in remission who have not received chemotherapy for at least 3 months may receive vaccines that contain live attenuated measles, mumps or rubella viruses (eg, MMR). Some forms of steroid therapy are not contraindications to immunization with live virus vaccines (for example, low to moderate doses for fewer than 2 weeks; every-other-day treatment regimens; and topical, intra-articular, and intrabursal administration). However, oral doses of approximately 20 mg of prednisone per day or topical doses likely to cause systemic effects contraindicate the use of live virus vaccines.

In persons with a family history of congenital immunodeficiency, oral polio vaccine is contraindicated until the immunocompetence of other household members is established. Although measles, mumps, and rubella vaccines contain live virus, they can be given to family members of immunocompromised patients since infection is not transmitted to others. Oral polio vaccine should not be used to immunize immunocompromised patients, their household contacts, or nursing personnel in close contact with such patients. Instead, enhanced-potency, inactivated polio vaccine is recom-

TABLE 1.2.   Misconceptions Concerning Contraindications to Adult
             Immunization

The following are *not* contraindications to vaccination:

1. Reaction to a previous vaccination consisting only of mild to moderate local tenderness, redness and/or swelling, or fever less than 40.5 °C
2. Mild acute illness with or without low-grade fever
3. Current antimicrobial therapy or convalescence from a recent illness
4. Household contact with a pregnant woman
5. Recent exposure to an infectious disease
6. Breast-feeding
7. Personal history of "allergies," including allergy to penicillin or other antibiotics, excluding anaphylactic reactions to neomycin (for example, combined measles, mumps, and rubella vaccine) or streptomycin (for example, oral polio vaccine)
8. Family history of "allergies," adverse reactions to vaccination, or seizures

mended for such immunocompromised patients and their household contacts.

Although there are few patients for whom specific vaccines are definitely contraindicated (*see* specific sections for individual vaccines), far more patients probably fail to receive needed vaccines because of misconceptions concerning contraindications to adult immunization. Some of the most common misconceptions are listed in Table 1.2.

Requirements for Patient Information, Recording, and Reporting of Adverse Events

The National Childhood Vaccine Injury Act (NCVIA) of 1986 requires the use of vaccine information statements for certain commonly used vaccines (MMR and polio vaccines, tetanus and diphtheria toxoids, and pertussis vaccine, which is not recommended for adults); mandates that information about the immunization given is permanently recorded; and requires reporting of adverse events associated with these vaccines.

Each patient or other responsible person should receive information about the risks of vaccines as well as their benefits in preventing disease in persons and in the larger community. Benefit and risk information should be presented in terms that are simple to understand. For the vaccines covered by the NCVIA, information in such materials is mandated to be presented in easily understood terms, must include all 10 points listed in Table 1.3, and must be given before immunization. Forms meeting these criteria were developed by the Centers for Disease Control and Prevention and are available through local and state health departments. These forms are written for children and their parents or guardians.

Each vaccine administration should be noted in the patient's medical record on a special immunization form (Appendix 7). This notation should include the type of vaccine; dose, site, and route of administration; name, address, and title of the person who gave the vaccine (required for NCVIA vaccines); date vaccine was given; manufacturer and lot number (required for NCVIA vaccines); and date the next dose is due. Health care providers who administer vaccines covered by the NCVIA are required by law to record this information permanently for these vaccines in the recipient's medical record or in an office log or file. These requirements apply to all patients, regardless of age, and to health care providers in both the private and public sectors. Recording such information for other vaccines is not required by law, but intelligent record keepers will do so anyway.

The patient should also be given a record containing information on the type of vaccine, the date given, the name of the doctor or clinic administering the vaccine, and the date the next dose is due. A prototype immunization record for the patient is shown in Appendix 8. Immunization record forms used in public clinics may differ from this format, but most are similar. These forms can be obtained from local or state health departments.

TABLE 1.3. **Information Required by Law to be Given to Vaccine Recipients before Immunization***

1. Frequency, severity, and potential long-term effects of the disease to be prevented by the vaccine
2. Symptoms or reactions to the vaccine that should be brought to the immediate attention of the health care provider
3. Precautionary measures to reduce the risk for any major adverse reactions to the vaccine that may occur
4. Early warning signs or symptoms that may be possible precursors to such major adverse reactions
5. A description of the manner in which to monitor such major adverse reactions, including a form on which reactions can be recorded to assist reporting information to appropriate authorities
6. A specification of when, how, and to whom any major adverse reaction should be reported
7. The contraindications to (and bases for delay of) the administration of the vaccine
8. Identification of the groups, categories, or characteristics of potential recipients of the vaccine who may be at significantly high risk for major adverse reaction to the vaccine compared with the general population
9. A summary of relevant Federal recommendations for a complete schedule of childhood immunizations; and the availability of the National Vaccine Injury Compensation Program
10. Such other relevant information as may be determined by the Secretary of Health and Human Services

* Applies to measles, mumps, rubella, pertussis, and polio vaccines, and tetanus and diphtheria toxoids.

Modern vaccines are generally safe, effective, and free from major side effects. However, adverse events have been reported after immunization with all vaccines, ranging from frequent, minor, local reactions to extremely rare, severe, systemic conditions such as paralysis associated with oral polio vaccine. Health care providers are required by the NCVIA to report specific events occurring within specified intervals after certain vaccinations. These are outlined in Appendix 9. Other adverse events that are serious or unusual should also be reported. All such reports should go to the Vaccine Adverse Events Reporting System (VAERS).The forms and instructions for this system are available in the *FDA Drug Bulletin* (Food and Drug Administration) and the *Physicians' Desk Reference* or by calling VAERS at 1-800-822-7967.

Vaccine Administration

The recommended route of administration for each vaccine is specified in the package insert. Care should be taken to ensure the appropriate route is used. Most adult vaccinations are given by intramuscular or subcutaneous injection. These injections are usually given in the anterior thigh in children or in the deltoid muscle in adults. The standard needle length is 5/8 inches, but for intramuscular administration of vaccine to patients who are obese, a 1- or 1.5-inch needle may be necessary to insure that the injection is truly intramuscular. The buttock is not recommended as a site for routine immunization. Studies with hepatitis B vaccine in adults have shown that its immunogenicity is significantly lower when injections are given in the buttock. This consideration also may apply to other vaccines. The buttock can be used for large-volume injections (for example, immune globulin), but care should be taken to give the injection in the upper, outer quadrant to avoid injury to the sciatic nerve.

Recommended doses vary for different vaccines but are typically 0.5 mL to 1.0 mL for subcutaneous or intramuscular injections and 0.1 mL to 0.2 mL for intradermal injections. The package inserts contain specific dosage information. The serologic response, clinical efficacy, and severity of adverse reactions from smaller doses of certain vaccines have not been studied adequately. Use of such smaller single doses or multiple doses to equal a full immunizing dose is not recommended.

Intradermal administration may be used for some vaccines, including booster parenteral typhoid, cholera, and pre-exposure human diploid cell rabies vaccine (rabies vaccine, adsorbed, should not be given intradermally). These injections are usually given in the volar surface of the forearm or over the deltoid area. Particular care should be taken to ensure that the

TABLE 1.4.   Guidelines for Spacing Live and Killed Antigen Administration

Antigen Combination	Recommended Minimum Interval between Doses
≥2 killed antigens	None; may be given simultaneously or at any interval between doses*
Killed and live antigens	None; may be given simultaneously or at any interval between doses†
≥2 live antigens	Four-week minimum interval if not administered simultaneously‡

* If possible, vaccines associated with local or systemic side effects (for example, cholera, typhoid, and plague vaccines) should be given on separate occasions to avoid accentuated reactions.
† Cholera vaccine with yellow fever vaccine is the exception. If time permits, these antigens should not be administered simultaneously, and at least 3 weeks should elapse between administration of yellow fever vaccine and cholera vaccine. If the vaccines must be given simultaneously or within 3 weeks of each other, the antibody response may not be optimal.
‡ The recent receipt of oral polio vaccine is not a contraindication to measles-mumps-rubella vaccine.
Source: General recommendations on immunizations. MMWR. 1994;43 (RR-1):1-39.

injection is not given subcutaneously, because this probably will reduce its effectiveness.

Minimum Intervals between Administration of Vaccines and Immune Globulin Preparations

Most widely used vaccines are safe and effective when given simultaneously (Table 1.4). This approach can be helpful in circumstances such as imminent exposure to several infectious diseases, preparation for foreign travel, or uncertainty about the patient's return for further doses of vaccine.

Guidelines for spacing live and killed antigen vaccines are given in Table 1.4. Killed vaccines generally can be administered simultaneously at separate sites. However, when vaccines commonly associated with more pronounced local or systemic side effects (for example, cholera and typhoid vaccines) are given simultaneously, the side effects theoretically could be accentuated. When practical, these vaccines should be given on separate occasions.

With the exception of cholera and yellow fever vaccines, inactivated and live attenuated virus vaccines can also be administered simultaneously at separate sites as long as the precautions that apply to each vaccine are followed.

Simultaneous administration of the most widely used live virus vaccines does not impair antibody responses or increase rates of adverse reactions. When feasible, live virus vaccines not administered on the same day should be given at least 1 month apart because of the theoretical concern that the immune response to one might be impaired if it is given within 1 month

TABLE 1.5. Guidelines for Spacing the Administration of Immune Globulin Preparations and Vaccines*

Administration	Recommended Minimum Interval between Doses
Simultaneous Immunobiologic Combination	
Immune globulin and killed antigen	None; may be given simultaneously at different sites or at any time between doses
Immune globulin and live antigen	Should generally not be given simultaneously[†]. If they must be given together, give at different sites and revaccinate or test for seroconversion after the interval recommended in Table 1.6 (for measles-mumps-rubella, measles-rubella, and monovalent measles vaccine)

Nonsimultaneous		
First	**Second**	
Immune globulin	Killed antigen	None
Killed antigen	Immune globulin	None
Immune globulin	Live antigen	Dose related[†,‡]
Live antigen	Immune globulin	2 weeks

*Blood products containing large amounts of immune globulin (such as serum immune globulin, specific immune globulins [eg, tetanus, hepatitis, B, etc.], intravenous immune globulin, whole blood, and packed red cells).

[†] Oral polio, yellow fever, and oral typhoid (Ty21a) vaccines are exceptions to these recommendations. These vaccines may be administered at any time before, after, or simultaneously with, an immune globulin-containing blood product without significantly decreasing the antibody response.

[‡] The duration of interference of immune globulin preparations with the immune response to the measles component of the measles-mumps-rubella, measles-rubella, and monovalent measles vaccine is dose related (see Table 1.6).

Source: General recommendations on immunization. MMWR. 1994;43 (RR-1):1-39.

of the other. However, recent receipt of oral polio virus is not a contraindication to administration of MMR.

Immune globulin and various disease-specific immune globulins contain antibodies that can interfere with the response to certain parenterally administered, live, attenuated virus vaccines (Table 1.5). Immune globulin preparations interact less with inactivated vaccines than with live vaccines. Therefore, administration of inactivated vaccines simultaneously or at any interval before or after receipt of immune globulins should not significantly impair a protective antibody response. The vaccine and immune globulin preparation should be given at different sites, and standard doses of the corresponding vaccine should be used. Increasing the vaccine dose volume or number of immunizations is not indicated.

Oral polio and yellow fever vaccines are not affected by administration of immune globulin or specific immune globulins at any time. Concurrent administration of immune globulin should not interfere with the immune response to oral typhoid vaccine, although published data are not available to corroborate this.

If administration of an immune globulin preparation becomes necessary because of imminent exposure to disease, MMR or its component vaccines can be given simultaneously with the immune globulin preparation, with the caveat that vaccine-induced immunity might be compromised. The vaccine should be administered at a site remote from that chosen for the immune globulin inoculation. Vaccination should be repeated after the interval recommended in Table 1.6, unless serologic testing indicates that specific antibodies were produced.

Because blood (for example, whole blood, packed red blood cells, plasma, and so on) and other antibody-containing blood products (for example, immune globulin, hepatitis B immunoglobulin, varicella zoster immunoglobulin, immune globulin intravenous, and so on) can diminish the immune response to MMR or its individual component vaccines, these vaccines should not be given after receipt of an immune globulin preparation before the interval recommended in Table 1.6. However, the postpartum vaccination of rubella-susceptible women with rubella or MMR vaccine should not be delayed because of receipt of anti-Rho(D) immune globulin (human) or any other blood product during the last trimester of pregnancy or at delivery. These women should be vaccinated immediately after delivery and, if possible, tested at least 3 months later to verify that immunity.

If administration of an immune globulin preparation becomes necessary after MMR or its individual component vaccines is given, interference can occur (Table 1.5). Usually, vaccine virus replication and stimulation of immunity occurs 1 or 2 weeks after vaccination. Thus, if the interval between administration of any of these vaccines and subsequent administration of an immune globulin preparation is less than 14 days, vaccination should be repeated after the interval recommended in Table 1.6, unless serologic testing indicates that antibodies were produced.

Products Available

A list of vaccines, toxoids, immune globulins, and their manufacturers and product names is included as Appendix 2. Because the number of manufacturers may change, the Center for Biologics Evaluation and Research of the Food and Drug Administration should be consulted for any new entries. Prices also are subject to change. The manufacturers can provide current prices.

Vaccine Storage and Handling

Some vaccines are stable, but others, including most live virus vaccines, are sensitive to heat and light. Instructions for storing and handling each vaccine are given in the package insert. Although some vaccines can or should be stored frozen, others (for example, tetanus and diphtheria toxoids, and hepatitis B vaccine) should never be frozen because freezing can cause aggregation and clumping of particles and lead to increased local reactions, decreased immunogenicity, or both.

Cost-Effectiveness and Cost-Benefit of Immunization

The first edition of the *Guide for Adult Immunization* cited Benjamin Franklin's aphorism that "an ounce of prevention is worth a pound of cure," thus giving prevention a cost-benefit ratio of 1:16. Interestingly, this figure is similar to the cost-benefit ratio (1:14.4) that was calculated for childhood MMR. In the past decade, attention has also been given to the cost-effectiveness and cost-benefit of adult immunization. Influenza and pneumococcal vaccines have received the most attention, and both have been determined to be cost-effective if given to elderly persons (65 years or older) and to younger persons with high-risk conditions. Hepatitis B vaccine is cost-effective for health care workers and other high-risk groups. The benefits in terms of reduced morbidity and mortality of universal childhood immunization with hepatitis B vaccine are comparable to those of other childhood vaccines. Previous recommendations for selective immunization of high-risk groups against hepatitis B were poorly implemented and did not reduce the incidence of hepatitis B; therefore, universal immunization of infants is now recommended. Both the cost of the vaccine, which is greater for adults than for children, and the difficulty in immunizing young adults who do not have regular contact with the health care system, have been deterrents to effective immunization of young adults. The high costs of controlling outbreaks of measles and rubella have been documented repeatedly, suggesting that even in the absence of a formal cost-effectiveness analysis, the benefits of vaccinating adults against these diseases may be substantial.

TABLE 1.6.   Suggested Intervals between Administration of Immune Globulin
            Preparations for Different Indications and Vaccines Containing
            Live Measles Virus*

Indications	Dose (Including mg IgG/kg)	Suggested Interval *months*
Washed red blood cells	10 mL/kg (negligible IgG/kg) IV	0
Tetanus prophylaxis (TIG)	250 units (~10 mg IgG/kg) IM	3
Hepatitis A prophylaxis (IG)		
Contact prophylaxis	0.02 mL/kg (3.3 mg IgG/kg) IM	3
International travel	0.06 mL/kg (9.9 mg IgG/kg) IM	
Hepatitis B prophylaxis (HBIG)	0.06 mL/kg (9.9 mg IgG/kg) IM	3
Reconstituted red blood cells	10 mL/kg (10 mg IgG/kg) IV	3
Rabies immune globulin (HRIG)	20 IU/kg (22 mg IgG/kg) IM	4
Varicella prophylaxis (VZIG)	125 units/10 kg (20-39 mg IgG/kg) IM (maximum 625 units)	5
Measles prophylaxis (IG)		
Normal contact	0.25 mL/kg (41 mg IgG/kg) IM	5
Immunocompromised contact	0.50 mL/kg (82 mg IgG/kg) IM	6
Packed red blood cells (Hct 65%)[†]	10 mL/kg (21–56 mg IgG/kg) IV	5–6
Whole blood (Hct 36%)[†]	10 mL/kg (38–100 mg IgG/kg) IV	6
Plasma/platelet products	10mL/kg (160 mg IgG/kg) IV	7
Replacement of humoral immune deficiencies (as IGIV)	160 mg/kg IV[‡]	7
	320 mg/kg IV[‡]	8
Treatment of:		
ITP[§] (as IGIV)	400 mg/kg IV	9
ITP[§] (as IGIV)	1000 mg/kg IV	10
Kawasaki disease (IGIV)	2 g/kg IV	11

* This table is not intended for purposes of determining the correct indications and dose for the use of immune globulin preparations. Unvaccinated persons may not be fully protected against measles during the entire interval and additional doses of immune globulin and/or measles vaccine may be indicated after measles exposure. The concentration of measles antibody in a particular immune globulin preparation may vary by lot. The rate of antibody clearance after receipt of an immune globulin preparation can also vary. The recommended intervals are extrapolated from an estimated half-life of 30 days for passively acquired antibody and an observed interference with the immune response to measles vaccine for as long as 5 months after a dose of 80 mg IgG/kg.

IV = intravenous; IM = intramuscular; Hct = hematocrit; IGIV = immune globulin, intravenous.
[†] Assumes a serum IgG concentration of 6 to 16 mg/mL.
[‡] Measles vaccination is recommended for children with HIV infection but is contraindicated in patients with congenital disorders of the immune system.
[§] Immune (idiopathic) thrombocytopenic purpura.
Source: General recommendations on immunization. MMWR. 1994;43 (RR-1):1-39.

2.

Implementation Strategies

Importance of Organized Programs for Vaccine Delivery

Despite the generally favorable attitudes of physicians toward vaccines for adults and evidence that vaccines are cost-effective, adult immunization is not widespread. Influenza, pneumococcal, and hepatitis B vaccines are especially underused. In the United States, nearly one half of elderly persons do not regard influenza as a threat to their health and think influenza vaccine is unnecessary. Even more elderly persons are unfamiliar with the danger of pneumococcal infections. Only about one third of high-risk persons receive influenza vaccine each year, and fewer than 20% have ever received pneumococcal vaccine. In Canada, the percentage of persons receiving influenza vaccine is only slightly higher than in the United States, and pneumococcal vaccine is rarely given.

An increasing fraction of office practices in general internal medicine are becoming computerized. Increased use of electronic billing practices will encourage this development and most physicians' offices will create an electronic database for the patients they treat. Although these systems will improve office administration and cash flow, their role in enhancing the delivery of preventive services has not been well developed. These data sets can be powerful tools to assess practice performance. The following example describes how use of such data can improve the delivery of influenza vaccine.

The central theme of this approach is the target-based or denominator-based concept whereby physicians view all of their patients as a population for whom certain services should be provided regularly. Such a concept is unfamiliar to most internists. Medical residencies generally stress the intensely personal, one-on-one interaction with patients, with the greatest emphasis placed on the patient encounter.

A population-based approach is different because it mandates that certain services, usually screening or preventive ones, be delivered to groups of patients and that progress in meeting these goals be monitored regularly. Three essential components of this target-based or denominator-based approach exist. The first is the accurate enumeration of patients in a prac-

TABLE 2.1.   Steps to Be Taken by Office Staff to Set Up and Use a Target-Based Approach to Deliver Influenza Vaccine to the Elderly

1. Generate an alphabetical list of all patients 65 years or older using computerized billing records
2. Ensure that the responsible physician reviews the list for accuracy
3. Determine the total number of patients—the total is the target for the practice
4. Enter the total on a simple poster that will allow monitoring of performance (Figure 1.)
5. Tally number of vaccinated persons as they receive vaccine
6. Monitor performance by plotting cumulative weekly influenza immunization rate

tice by name, address, age, and principal diagnosis; the second is the establishment of a target (patient group) for a particular service such as annual influenza immunization for all persons 65 years and older; and the third is a means to record delivered services so a performance rate can be calculated.

This approach is particularly useful for ensuring that elderly persons receive influenza vaccines annually; it is important because of the proportional relation between increased age and higher rates of morbidity and mortality from influenza infection. Thus, all persons 65 years or older are targets for yearly influenza immunization. One important logistic hurdle in delivering influenza vaccine in the office setting is that vaccines are given during a 2- or 3-month period, and eligible patients may not be scheduled to see their physicians during that time. To achieve high immunization rates, physicians must develop proactive initiatives to immunize all eligible patients and not only those persons who have a visit scheduled when influenza vaccine is being given in the office.

From 1988 to 1991, internists and family practitioners in private practices in Monroe County, New York, participated in a series of demonstration studies to determine whether a target-based approach could increase influenza immunizations in elderly persons. These studies clearly show that immunization performance can be increased substantially after physicians are made aware of targets within their practice and are given a simple means to monitor their performance.

Table 2.1 lists the procedures necessary to implement this concept. The first step is the most important and requires an alphabetical enumeration of all patients 65 years or older in the practice. This usually can be done electronically by office staff or by the practice's billing service. For group practices, the lists should be physician-specific. Once prepared, the list should be reviewed by the responsible physician to determine whether patients on the list are still in the practice. This list becomes the target population for the physician. The total number of patients is inserted onto a poster or chart

FIGURE 1

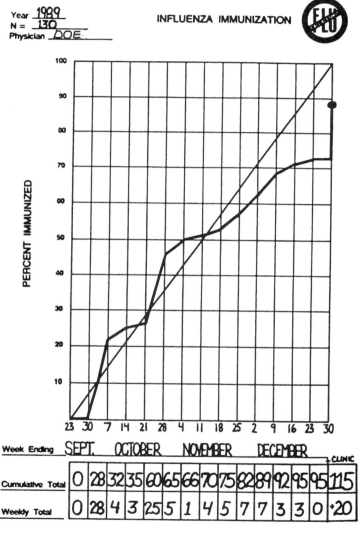

(Figure 1). As persons in the target group are vaccinated, they are listed on the form. Marking off vaccinees from the target list by the nurse or the physician administering the immunizations creates a list of persons who are not immunized. Persons refusing vaccination are also noted. Each week, the cumulative fraction of the target patients who received influenza vaccine is recorded on the chart so the physician and his or her office staff are always aware of their performance. Practices may want to call or send cards to persons not scheduled for appointments when influenza vaccine is given. The key factor is that influenza vaccine be offered in a positive manner to all eligible persons. The two essential components of this approach are (1) a clear, unambiguous definition of a target population and (2) a simple system whereby progress in immunizing these persons can be monitored.

This approach was used in more than 100 group and solo practices; more than 70% of elderly persons received influenza immunization in Monroe County. The highest immunization rates were in those practices with the following characteristics: active physician support; use of a physician-specific monitoring system; involvement of the office staff.

This approach can be used for most vaccines. For example, sorting the patients in a practice for chronic cardiac or pulmonary diseases or both identifies another target population for influenza and pneumococcal vaccines. This technique can be integrated into other office-based approaches, such as chart and postcard reminders, and can be used to measure performance in the delivery of any preventive service such as annual clinical breast examination and mammography for all eligible women.

Physicians and other health care providers who care for patients in other settings must be concerned with adult immunization. Hospitals are important sites for immunization. In outpatient clinics and inpatient units, organized approaches for offering influenza and pneumococcal vaccines can lead to immunization rates of more than 50% to 70%. Such programs focus efforts on patients at substantial risk for these two diseases; two thirds of patients hospitalized for pneumococcal infections were hospitalized within the previous 5 years, and 25% or more of elderly patients admitted for influenza-associated respiratory conditions were discharged previously during the immunization season immediately preceding the outbreak period. Emergency rooms can also play an important role in influenza and pneumococcal vaccination, especially for persons who have no other source of routine medical care.

Hospitals also have an important role in immunizing adults against other vaccine-preventable diseases. Although prenatal screening for rubella antibody has become routine, greater efforts are needed to ensure that pregnant women who are not immune are given rubella vaccine after they deliver. Routine serologic screening of all pregnant women for hepatitis B is recommended to identify carriers of the virus. Newborn infants of carriers can be given hepatitis B immune globulin and hepatitis B vaccine. Implementing this requires a well-organized approach to prevention that involves many types of physicians. Similarly, ensuring that health care workers are also protected against hepatitis B, rubella, measles, and other vaccine-preventable diseases (especially influenza) requires an organized approach.

In other settings, immunization programs may require different approaches. For example, health maintenance organizations and other managed health care providers often pay greater attention to preventive measures and have information systems that facilitate organized programs for vaccine delivery. The American College Health Association now recommends that all students show records of immunity against measles, mumps, rubella, tetanus, and diphtheria. Some colleges have successfully implemented these recommendations by requiring such evidence before students enroll, before they are given grade reports, or before transcripts of their records are issued. Increases in hepatitis B vaccination have occurred recently among health care workers largely as a result of Occupational Safety and Health Association regulations.

These examples and many others provide convincing evidence that adult immunization can be successful if vaccination programs are well organized and efficiently administered. Nonetheless, such programs have not become widespread. Better vaccination strategies, not simply better vaccines, will be required if substantial improvements in adult immunization will be made.

3.

Immunizations for
Healthy Adults

Adolescents and Young Adults

Tetanus and Diphtheria

Most adolescents and young adults receive a three-dose primary series of tetanus and diphtheria toxoids (usually in combination with pertussis vaccine) during early childhood. The pediatric immunization schedule calls for diphtheria-pertussis-tetanus boosters at age 15 months and at 4 to 6 years and a tetanus-diphtheria (Td) toxoid booster at age 16 years. Others may have been immunized when they were students in elementary or secondary schools. Current state immunization requirements for school children are given in Appendix 4. A history of recent military service, travel, and special occupations may provide clues regarding previous immunization. If there is doubt about completion of a primary series, two doses (0.5 mL each) of combined Td toxoid should be given intramuscularly at least 4 weeks apart, followed by a third dose 6 to 12 months later. Although tetanus toxoid is available as a single immunogen, the combined Td toxoid should be used to enhance protection against both diseases.

Measles, Mumps, and Rubella

Young adults should be immune to measles, mumps, and rubella. Because of outbreaks in colleges and other schools, the Centers for Disease Control's Advisory Committee on Immunization Practices endorsed a two-dose measles schedule for children and selected adults in 1989. The second dose is not a booster, because the primary response is thought to provide long-term protection. The second dose is intended to immunize the approximately 5% of persons who do not respond to the first dose. The overall epidemiologic strategy is to achieve universal immunization with the first dose at 15 months and the second dose with entry into kindergarten or the first grade. Some states have stipulated receipt of the second dose of measles vaccine at a later age, such as entry into middle school or junior high school. Young adults who are attending college or who are at high risk for contracting measles (for example, if they are health care workers) should have proof of receipt of two doses of measles vaccine or have serologic or clinical evidence of immunity. The second dose of measles vaccine should be given for protection against measles, mumps, and rubella. All other young adults should have received at least one dose of measles, mumps, and rubella vaccine (MMR). As the current population of children enters adolescence, all persons in this age group will be required to have two doses of measles vaccine.

Women of childbearing age must be assured of immunity against rubella. Rubella vaccine should be given unless there is laboratory evidence of immunity or a record of vaccination after the first birthday. Susceptible women of childbearing age should not be vaccinated during pregnancy; instead, they should be vaccinated immediately after delivery. Combined MMR vaccine is preferred if uncertainty exists about immunity to more than one of these diseases. No increased risk for adverse reactions is associated with MMR vaccination in persons already immune to measles, mumps, or rubella.

Influenza

Influenza vaccination should be considered for young adults who provide essential community services, including health care workers who are at increased risk for acquiring influenza and transmitting it to high-risk patients. The vaccine may also be given to young adults at increased risk for exposure (for example, military personnel or college students living in dormitories). Influenza vaccine may also be given to anyone who wishes to reduce the likelihood of contracting influenza.

Twenty-Five to Sixty-Four Years

Tetanus and Diphtheria

All adults should have completed a primary series of immunization with tetanus and diphtheria toxoids. Those who have been partially immunized need only to complete the three-dose Td schedule. The Task Force on Adult Immunization supports two booster options: the traditional recommendation that Td boosters be given every 10 years throughout life; or, a single Td booster given at age 50 years for persons who have completed the full pediatric series, including the teenage/young adult booster.

Measles, Mumps, and Rubella

Adults born before 1957 may be considered immune to measles and mumps. For those who are younger, a documented physician's diagnosis of measles and mumps, or laboratory evidence of infection, is acceptable evidence of immunity. In addition, most adults can be considered immune if they have a dated record of immunization. However, persons vaccinated against measles between 1963 and 1967 may have received inactivated vaccine and should receive a single dose of live vaccine to prevent the development of atypical measles. Also, persons who received inactivated measles vaccine followed within 5 months by live vaccine should be immunized again. A clinical diagnosis of rubella is nonspecific, and proof of immunity requires serologic confirmation or a record of rubella vaccination. Susceptible women who are pregnant should receive rubella vaccine after delivery. The combined MMR vaccine should be used for persons who may be susceptible to more than one of these diseases.

Influenza and Pneumococcal Infections

Healthy adults younger than 65 years are not at increased risk for complications of influenza virus infection. However, those who provide essential community services, including health care personnel who are at increased risk for exposure to influenza or of transmitting infection to others, should be vaccinated. Influenza vaccine can also be given to anyone who wishes to reduce the risk for contracting influenza.

Pneumococcal vaccine is indicated for persons younger than 65 years who have risk factors for acquiring invasive pneumococcal disease. Approximately one third of persons 50 to 64 years old have conditions for which they should receive pneumococcal vaccine and annual influenza immunization. **The Task Force on Adult Immunization strongly recommends that age 50 years be established as a time for review of preventive health measures, with special emphasis on evaluating the need for pneumococcal vaccine, annual influenza immunization, and Td primary or booster immunization.**

Other Vaccines

In addition to the vaccines recommended above, adults in all age groups should be questioned about their lifestyles, occupations, and any special circumstances that warrant additional vaccines. For example, all persons at high risk for infection because they are intravenous drug users or have multiple sex partners (defined as more than one partner every 6 months) should receive hepatitis B vaccine.

Sixty-Five Years and Older

Elderly persons are susceptible to development of a number of infectious diseases, especially those of the lower respiratory tract. Despite advances in medical care, pneumonia and influenza remain the fifth leading cause of death in persons in this age group. Several factors may be responsible. For some persons, environmental circumstances such as institutional living may increase the likelihood of infection, particularly during influenza outbreaks. Decreasing cardiac and pulmonary function are also important. Aging itself is associated with a decrease in certain host-defense mechanisms, although these changes affect cell-mediated more than humoral immunity and have little effect on granulocyte or monocyte function.

All persons 65 years and older should receive both pneumococcal vaccine and annual influenza vaccine regardless of health status. Those who receive pneumococcal vaccine before age 65 years because they have certain risk factors should be considered for reimmunization at age 65, provided that at least 6 years have passed since the first dose of pnuemococcal vaccine was given.

Influenza

Outbreaks of influenza generally occur each year. Reports of excess pneumonia and influenza deaths underestimate the overall mortality rate associated with influenza because as many as two thirds of these deaths are reported as being due to other causes, particularly cardiovascular diseases. The effect of influenza is most severe among elderly persons, who account for 80% to 90% of all influenza-associated deaths. Approximately 90% of elderly persons who die have recognized underlying high-risk conditions, but deaths also occur among those who appear to be healthy. In addition, elderly persons are hospitalized more often for pneumonia and influenza during epidemic periods.

Protection against influenza virus infections correlates best with a serum antihemagglutinin antibody titer of 1:40 or more. As a group, healthy elderly persons have reduced mean antibody responses compared with those in younger adults. These differences may reflect the decreased immunoresponsiveness of elderly persons or higher pre-existing antibody titers that can blunt the antihemagglutinin response to influenza vaccine. Nonetheless, the antibody responses of many elderly persons are similar to those seen in younger adults.

The clinical efficacy of influenza vaccination to reduce deaths among elderly persons has not been shown in a randomized, controlled trial. However, uncontrolled studies have shown vaccination to be 70% to 100% protective against death caused by influenza. Furthermore, other studies have shown that influenza vaccination reduces rates of hospitalization among elderly persons with greater risk factors and is cost-effective.

All elderly persons, not just those with high-risk conditions, should receive influenza vaccine each year. It is the responsibility of physicians to educate their patients about this need. Once this is done, and influenza vaccine is offered and accepted, elderly persons may expect and even ask for influenza vaccine in subsequent years, thus assuring up-to-date protection against this serious disease.

Pneumococcal Infections

Epidemiologic data are more difficult to obtain for pneumococcal infections than for influenza. Recent community studies of pneumococcal bacteremia have documented an overall incidence of 15 to 19 cases per 100 000 persons each year. In persons 65 years and older, the incidence of pneumococcal bacteremia increases to 50 cases per 100 000 persons each year. Pneumococcal infections continue to be the leading cause of adult community-acquired pneumonia requiring hospitalization. Among elderly patients with pneumococcal bacteremia, case-fatality rates remain high despite administration of appropriate antimicrobial therapy. Although the annual incidence of serious pneumococcal infection among elderly persons appears to be stable, the continued high case-fatality rate and the increasing problem of antibiotic-resistant strains of pneumococci are compelling reasons to provide prophylaxis with pneumococcal vaccine.

Limited information on the antibody responses of elderly persons to pneumococcal vaccination is available. Older persons may have lower antibody titers to certain pneumococcal types (for example, types 3 and 8) before and 2 weeks after immunization compared with titers in younger persons. However, the mean levels of antibody in elderly persons usually increase at least 10 times after immunization.

The efficacy of pneumococcal vaccination in preventing pneumococcal pneumonia in elderly persons has not been shown in a modern randomized, controlled trial. However, case-control and epidemiologic studies have shown that the aggregate efficacy of pneumococcal vaccination is approximately 55% to 70% in preventing pneumococcal bacteremia in the elderly, although it may be less effective in those who are immunocompromised.

Limited data on the persistence of antibody levels in the elderly indicate that titers decrease after 6 years. Clinical trials showed that revaccination with pneumococcal vaccine after 6 years is not associated with an increased risk for adverse reactions. Revaccination should be done after 6 years for those at highest risk for acquiring fatal infection (asplenic patients) and those with medical conditions associated with rapid antibody loss, such as those receiving dialysis. Insufficient data on revaccination of healthy elderly persons preclude a precise recommendation.

Tetanus and Diphtheria

Almost all cases of tetanus and most of the handful of diphtheria cases in the United States occur in persons who have never completed a primary series of vaccination for these diseases. For tetanus, more than one half of reported cases occur in persons 60 years and older. Many of these cases follow injuries that are not normally associated with tetanus. Serologic studies indicate that 40% or more of elderly persons lack adequate levels of Td antitoxins. Despite declining immunoresponsiveness, elderly persons can still mount a strong antibody response to Td toxoids. Physicians should ensure that all their elderly patients have completed a primary vaccination series. Those who are partially immunized need only complete the three-dose Td schedule. The Task Force on Adult Immunization supports two booster options: the traditional recommended Td boosters every 10 years throughout life, and a single mid-life Td booster at age 50 for persons who have completed a full primary series.

Other Vaccines

In addition to giving vaccines that are routinely recommended, physicians should ask all older adults about their lifestyles, occupations, and special circumstances, such as impending travel, that may prompt consideration of other vaccines.

4.

Immunizations for Special Groups of Patients

Pregnant Women

All unnecessary medications or procedures that might jeopardize the fetus should be avoided during pregnancy. The risks associated with vaccination, however, are largely theoretical, and the advantages usually outweigh the potential risks for adverse reactions. This is especially so when exposure to infection is likely, if the infection is particularly dangerous to the mother or fetus, and if the vaccine is unlikely to cause harm. Furthermore, newer information continues to confirm the safety of vaccines given inadvertently during pregnancy.

In the future, immunization of pregnant women may be indicated to ensure the transfer of maternal antibody to the fetus, as with tetanus. Whenever a vaccine or a toxoid is indicated during pregnancy, waiting until the second or third trimester is reasonable, although no risk from earlier immunization has been proved. Live virus vaccines should be avoided unless specifically indicated. The benefits of preventing disease during pregnancy clearly outweigh concerns about the safety of vaccines or immune globulins under special circumstances, such as exposure to rabies, hepatitis A, or hepatitis B.

Women of childbearing age should be immunized against poliomyelitis, measles, mumps, rubella, tetanus, and diphtheria before becoming pregnant. Assessment of immunity begins with a history of previous illnesses and immunizations. However, many adults will not have reliable records or memory of childhood illnesses and immunizations. This is particularly important for rubella because of the consequences of infection for the developing fetus. A history of maternal rubella or undocumented immunization is often unreliable and cannot be accepted as proof of immunity. In addition, hepatitis B virus (HBV) can cause subclinical infections, and pregnant women can be carriers of the virus without knowing it, thus risking perinatal infection of their newborn infants. Because both rubella and hepatitis B pose serious risks for the fetus and newborn, all pregnant women should be screened for rubella antibody and hepatitis B surface antigen.

Hepatitis A

If hepatitis A occurs during pregnancy, an increased risk for severe maternal infection, abortion, and prematurity exists. Some women who are exposed to hepatitis A will be immune because of previous infection. If she is not immune, the pregnant woman should receive immune globulin (0.02 mL/kg administered intramuscularly) as soon as possible, preferably within 1 week of exposure. A killed hepatitis A vaccine is expected to be licensed in the near future.

Hepatitis B

In a pregnant woman, HBV infection can result in severe disease and fetal loss for the mother, and chronic infection for the newborn. Pregnancy should not be considered a contraindication for hepatitis B vaccination of women in high-risk groups.

All pregnant women should have routine prenatal screening for hepatitis B surface antigen (HBsAg). Those who are seronegative and at high risk for becoming infected with HBV should be vaccinated. Mothers who are long-term carriers of HBsAg, particularly those who are positive for the e antigen, are likely to transmit infection to their infants during the perinatal period. The combination of hepatitis B vaccine and hepatitis B immune globulin given to newborn infants is 90% to 95% effective in preventing perinatal transmission of hepatitis B (Table 8.3).

Immune Globulin

The indications for using immune globulin, intravenous immune globulin, and specific immune globulins (for example, tetanus immune globulin) in pregnant women are the same as those for women who are not pregnant. These preparations are safe and not associated with added risk for adverse reactions.

Influenza and Pneumococcal Infections

Influenza and pneumococcal vaccines are indicated for pregnant women with underlying high-risk conditions, but they are not routinely recommended for those who are otherwise healthy. Although experience is limited, no evidence exists that either vaccine will harm the fetus. The vaccines can be given simultaneously at different sites.

Measles, Mumps, and Rubella

Because of the theoretical risk to the fetus, live virus vaccines generally are not given to pregnant women or to those who are likely to become pregnant within 3 months. Women born before 1957 are likely to have acquired natural immunity to measles and mumps. The immediate postpartum peri-od is a good time to administer measles vaccine to younger women who lack documentation of vaccination on or after their first birthdays, physi-cian-diagnosed measles, or laboratory evidence of immunity. The combined measles, mumps, and rubella (MMR) vaccine should be used because such women also may be susceptible to mumps or rubella.

Because occurrence of measles during pregnancy increases the risk for premature labor and spontaneous abortion, a susceptible pregnant woman exposed to measles should be given immune globulin intramuscularly with-in 6 days of exposure. She should then be given MMR vaccine after delivery, at least 5 months after receipt of immune globulin.

The wild-type mumps virus can infect the placenta and fetus but does not appear to cause congenital malformations. The mumps vaccine virus has been shown to infect the placenta, but it has not been isolated from fetal tissues from susceptible women who were vaccinated and who then had an abortion. Immune globulin is not effective for post-exposure prophylaxis of mumps and is not recommended.

The fetal risk from maternal rubella is much greater than that from measles or mumps. If a woman is exposed to rubella during the first 20 weeks of pregnancy, a serologic test should be performed to determine immunity. If she is found to be susceptible, she should be retested 2 to 4 weeks later and, if infection has occurred, counseled regarding her options. If rubella is con-tracted during the first 20 weeks of pregnancy, fetal or early neonatal death will occur in 15% to 20% of cases. Among infants who survive, 20% to 50% will have evidence of congenital rubella syndrome (for example, cataracts, deafness, and congenital heart disease). If an exposed pregnant woman decides not to terminate her pregnancy if she contracts rubella, immune globulin can be given in the same timing and dosage as for measles, although current evidence has not proved that this treatment is protective.

Preventing fetal infection and congenital rubella syndrome are the pri-mary objectives of rubella immunization. Unlike measles, a history of rubel-la is not a reliable indicator of immunity. Serologic screening is not neces-sary before vaccinating a woman of childbearing age who is not pregnant. She should be advised not to become pregnant for 3 months because of the theoretical risk to the fetus. If she becomes pregnant or is already pregnant and is inadvertently given rubella vaccine, the experience among more than 300 such women has not shown a detectable risk for vaccine-associated mal-formations.

Poliomyelitis

Poliovirus infection can cause fetal loss during early pregnancy and congenital paralytic infection during late pregnancy. However, successful immunization programs have eliminated illness due to wild poliovirus in the United States, and global eradication of poliomyelitis is a major public health goal of the 1990s. Therefore, except for rare localized outbreaks in unimmunized groups, the risk for poliomyelitis is related mainly to foreign travel to areas where wild polioviruses still exist. Pregnant women need not be immunized against poliomyelitis unless they are exposed to a risk factor for the disease.

Two vaccines are available to prevent poliomyelitis: enhanced-potency inactivated polio vaccine and live oral polio vaccine. For pregnant women at high risk for exposure and who have completed a primary series of polio vaccination more than 10 years previously, a single, one-time booster dose of enhanced-potency inactivated polio vaccine is recommended to ensure an adequate response to all three poliovirus antigens. For an unimmunized pregnant woman at high risk for exposure to poliovirus infection, two doses of enhanced-potency inactivated polio vaccine should be given at intervals of 1 to 2 months. If fewer than 4 weeks are available for immunization and immediate protection is needed, a single dose of oral polio vaccine may be given. The remaining doses of the primary series for either vaccine should be given at the appropriate intervals if the woman is still at increased risk.

Tetanus and Diphtheria

Pregnant women who have not been immunized against tetanus and diphtheria should receive two doses of the combined tetanus and diphtheria toxoid given 4 to 8 weeks apart, preferably during the second or third trimesters. This should be followed by a third dose 6 to 12 months later to complete the primary series. If the primary series was not completed, or if the woman was immunized more than 10 years earlier, one or two booster doses of combined tetanus and diphtheria toxoid should be given as indicated. The protection of the newborn infant that is conferred by placental transfer of maternal antibody will persist for approximately 6 months.

Varicella Zoster

Pregnant women in whom primary varicella develops may have an increased risk for serious complications (for example, pneumonia and premature labor) compared with other women. Susceptible women who are exposed to varicella zoster may be given varicella zoster immune globulin, which may prevent or modify serious maternal illness, but no evidence exists that it will prevent intrauterine infection. Acyclovir should be reserved for severe maternal varicella infection in which the potential benefit justifies the potential risk to the fetus. Infants born to mothers in whom varicella develops within 5 days before or 48 hours after delivery should receive varicella zoster immune globulin to reduce the likelihood of serious or fatal neonatal varicella infection. A live attenuated varicella vaccine will soon be licensed and susceptible women of childbearing age will be targeted for immunization.

Yellow Fever

Yellow fever vaccine contains live attenuated virus, but it is not known to be teratogenic. If a pregnant woman must travel to an area where yellow fever is known to be prevalent, immunization with live attenuated yellow fever vaccine should be considered. The risk for disease is very small for most tourists, and no American traveler is known to have contracted yellow fever in the past 50 years. Because yellow fever immunization is a requirement for entry into certain countries, the physician who elects not to immunize a pregnant woman should provide her with an explanatory letter.

Women Who Are Breast-feeding

Breast-feeding does not adversely effect the response to immunization and is not a contraindication for any of the currently recommended vaccines.

Family Member Exposure

When members of family groups develop certain transmissible illnesses, vaccines, antibiotics, or immune globulin preparations can be used to protect family members or other close household contacts.

Haemophilus influenzae Type b

Haemophilus influenzae type b vaccines are not indicated for adults or children in contact with a family member who has meningitis caused by *H. influenzae* type b infection (unless the uninfected child is younger than 4 years and has not previously been immunized). In households with a susceptible child younger than 4 years, rifampin prophylaxis should be given to all contacts, including adults, with the exception of pregnant women.

Hepatitis A

Hepatitis A is transmitted primarily by the fecal-oral route. Immune globulin will modify or prevent illness and should be given to other susceptible family members once the index case is diagnosed. Casual contact with a person with hepatitis A that occurs outside the household or does not include sharing food or a bed is not an indication for immune globulin prophylaxis.

Hepatitis B

Hepatitis B presents a risk for serious disease within families. If a family member has acute or chronic hepatitis B, his or her sexual partner and others with intimate contact (especially infants younger than 12 months) should be treated with one dose of hepatitis B immune globulin and started on a three-dose series of hepatitis B vaccine unless they are known to be immune. If household contact with a chronic hepatitis B carrier has been prolonged, testing family members for antibody to hepatitis B antigen (anti-HBs) and HBsAg will identify those already immune or who have become carriers.

Influenza

In families in which one member has a high-risk condition, the high-risk person and healthy family members should be vaccinated each fall. If an unimmunized healthy family member acquires an influenza-like illness during a community outbreak of type A influenza, he or she should begin treatment with rimantadine (or amantadine) to prevent transmission of infection within the household, and unimmunized family members with high-risk conditions should be vaccinated and given rimantadine (or amantadine) for 14 days.

Meningococcal Infections

Antimicrobial prophylaxis with rifampin, ciprofloxacin, or ceftriaxone is indicated for persons with close contact with a person with meningococcal meningitis (the index case). In closed populations, if the index case of meningitis was caused by serogroups A, C, Y, or W-135, meningococcal vaccine may also be effective because one half of secondary cases of disease occur more than 5 days after the primary case.

Poliomyelitis

When children are given oral polio vaccine, adults in the household who have not been adequately immunized incur a small risk for contracting vaccine-associated paralytic poliomyelitis. Because of the importance of ensuring prompt and complete immunization of children, and the rarity of vaccine-associated disease in persons in contact with vaccinated persons, children should be given oral polio vaccine regardless of the vaccination status of adult household members unless these persons are known to be immunocompromised. The responsible adult should be informed of the small risk involved and of precautions to be taken, such as hand washing after changing diapers. If strong assurance is received that full immunization of the child will not be jeopardized or unduly delayed, an acceptable alternative is to give at least two doses (4 to 8 weeks apart) of enhanced-potency inactivated polio vaccine to previously unimmunized adults before giving oral polio vaccine to the child. If the adult was previously partially immunized with one or more doses of oral polio vaccine, either oral polio vaccine or enhanced-potency inactivated polio vaccine can be given to complete the primary series. The child can be given oral polio vaccine at the same time.

Rubella

If rubella occurs in a family with a woman who is in the first 20 weeks of pregnancy, she should be tested immediately for rubella antibody. If she is not immune and is later shown by serologic testing to have become infected, she should be advised about the risk for congenital damage and counseled regarding her options.

Varicella Zoster

Susceptible family contacts of persons in whom primary varicella (chickenpox) or herpes zoster (shingles) develop do not need treatment unless these contacts are immunocompromised or pregnant. In this instance, varicella zoster immune globulin can be considered, depending on the severity of the underlying disease.

Environmental Situations

In certain environmental situations, increased risks of exposure to vaccine-preventable diseases exist. In these settings, immunizations other than those routinely recommended may be indicated.

Residents of Nursing Homes

All residents and staff of nursing homes should be immunized with influenza vaccine each year. If immunization rates exceed 80%, outbreaks of influenza are unlikely to occur. In nursing home influenza outbreaks, attack rates of 25% to 50% have been reported, and case-fatality rates among patients have reached 30%. To achieve high vaccination rates, influenza vaccine must be offered to residents as part of routine medical care; otherwise, the administrative burden of requiring written consent from relatives usually reduces immunization rates. When an influenza outbreak occurs, effective management includes immediate updating of influenza vaccination for residents and staff. If the outbreak is caused by type A influenza virus, rimantadine/amantadine chemoprophylaxis and chemotherapy of residents may provide additional protection for persons at high risk.

By age and underlying condition, most nursing home residents should receive pneumococcal vaccine. The need for a primary Td series or Td booster also should be assessed.

Residents of Institutions for the Mentally Retarded

Because of frequent exposure to blood and blood-contaminated fluids through bites and contact with open skin lesions, saliva, and other contaminated body secretions, residents in institutions for the mentally retarded are at increased risk for hepatitis B (in serosurveys, 30% to 80% have evidence of HBV infection). Residents of such institutions should be screened on entry, and those found to be susceptible should be vaccinated with hepatitis B vaccine. Because of the high prevalence of infection in such institutions, serologic screening of long-term residents before vaccination is probably cost-effective.

Prison Inmates

Serologic evidence of HBV infection can be found in 10% to 80% of male prisoners. Prisoners should be screened for HBsAg and anti-HBs. Those who are found to be susceptible should be immunized with hepatitis B vaccine. Hepatitis B vaccine will provide protection not only during the time in prison but also after the prisoner is released, when the risk for acquiring infection may be greater. Prisoners should also have routine immunizations reviewed and updated when indicated.

Homeless Persons

Few data are available on the vaccine needs of homeless persons. However, it is reasonable to assume that many will need primary or booster Td toxoid immunization, MMR (if they are younger adults), influenza, and pneumococcal vaccines. In addition, some may require hepatitis B vaccination. It is important that the need for vaccines not be overlooked whenever homeless persons are seen in emergency rooms or in other clinical settings.

Occupational Groups

College Students

College students are at risk for several vaccine-preventable infections because of their age-group susceptibility, importation of disease after foreign travel, and crowding in dormitories. Outbreaks of measles, rubella, and mumps have occurred on college campuses. These outbreaks have often been difficult and costly to control. The American College Health Association recommends that all colleges and universities adopt prematriculation immunization requirements for entering students. Several states have laws that require colleges to document the immunization status of their students.

Measles: The risk for serious illness and death due to measles is higher in young adults than in children. Among college students born after 1956, approximately 10% are not immune. Students should be given measles vaccine unless they can provide proof of immunization (two doses) after their first birthdays, physician-diagnosed disease, or laboratory evidence of immunity. Because measles outbreaks have occurred on college campuses, current policy is to revaccinate students of colleges and other institutions of higher learning who previously received one dose of measles vaccine. Repeated vaccination of those already immune causes no increase in adverse reactions. Excluding pregnancy by history and warning of the theoretical risks of vaccination during pregnancy are sufficient precautions. Because students might also be susceptible to mumps or rubella, MMR vaccine should be used. Because many outbreaks in college communities are caused by importation of measles virus from foreign countries, all students born after 1956 who travel to foreign countries where the risk of exposure is significant should be given measles vaccine (preferably MMR) unless they have already completed the two-dose schedule. Control measures for measles outbreaks in colleges should include revaccination of all students and younger staff who have received only one dose of measles vaccine.

Rubella: Universal immunization against rubella is recommended for college students unless they are known to be immune by documented vaccination or laboratory evidence of immunity. Without such evidence, serologic testing for rubella antibody is not necessary before MMR vaccine is given. Women who are pregnant should not be given MMR or rubella vaccines. Those who have been vaccinated should avoid becoming pregnant for 3 months after immunization.

Mumps: Because the two-dose measles schedule is almost always carried out with the MMR vaccine, college-age students are well immunized against mumps. For college students who have not previously received a mumps vaccine, a single dose of MMR or mumps monovalent vaccine is recommended.

Tetanus and Diphtheria: All adults, including college students, should have received routine primary immunization with combined tetanus and diphtheria toxoid during childhood including a Td booster at age 16. If this has not been done, a primary series should be completed. As an equivalent alternative to the current recommendations that all adults receive Td boosters every 10 years, the Task Force on Adult Immunization recommends a single Td booster at age 50 years for those who have completed a primary series including a teenage/young adult Td booster.

Hepatitis B: Hepatitis B vaccination should be considered strongly for all college students. Serologic screening before vaccination is not cost-effective because of the low prevalence of disease.

Poliomyelitis: Most college students have already received at least a three-dose primary series of oral polio vaccine. However, for students who have completed a primary series and who plan to travel to areas where wild polioviruses are endemic, a one-time extra dose of oral polio vaccine or enhanced-potency inactivated polio vaccine should be given. For those not previously immunized, a primary series of enhanced-potency inactivated polio vaccine should be given, the first two doses administered 4 to 8 weeks apart, followed by a third dose 6 to 12 months later. If there is time for only one dose, either oral polio vaccine or enhanced-potency inactivated polio vaccine can be used.

Meningococcal Infections: Routine immunization of college students with meningococcal vaccine is not recommended because of the low frequency of meningococcal infections in the United States. However, during outbreaks caused by serogroups represented in the vaccine, meningococcal vaccination should be considered as an adjunct to chemoprophylaxis with rifampin, ciprofloxacin, or ceftriaxone. Meningococcal vaccine should also be considered for students traveling to countries recognized as having high rates of meningococcal disease.

Health Care Workers

Health care workers are at particular risk for acquiring several vaccine-preventable diseases. Transmission of hepatitis B and influenza from patients to health care workers is frequent, and infection can be transmitted then to other patients. Rubella and measles have been transmitted both to and from health care workers and patients, sometimes with significant health care costs and potential legal consequences. A federal standard was issued in 1991 mandating that hepatitis B vaccine be made available to all at-risk health care personnel at the employer's expense. These regulations have accelerated and broadened the use of hepatitis B vaccine in health care workers. However, acceptance of the other vaccines by health care workers has been poor.

Hepatitis B: The risk for acquiring hepatitis B by health care workers is directly proportional to the degree of exposure to blood or blood products. Serologic evidence of previous HBV infection is 2 to 10 times more common in health care workers than in the community at large and increases with the level of disease in the community and the duration of exposure. The risk for infection is approximately 4% to 5% per decade of continued exposure to blood. Health care workers who are positive for anti-HBs outnumber those who are chronic HBV carriers (HBsAg positive) by approximately 20 to 1. Among health care workers, the highest rates of serologic markers for HBV infection are found among surgeons, oral surgeons, pathologists, and dialysis and certain laboratory personnel. Lower rates occur among pediatricians, internists, anesthesiologists, and family practitioners. In medical and surgical residents, the highest rates of acquiring HBV infection occur during the early years of training and decrease after years of experience and with decreased exposure. Health care workers with patient contact but no exposure to blood (for example, psychiatrists and social workers) are not at increased risk for acquiring HBV infection.

In most instances, transmission of HBV infection is not recognized. Only one third of HBV-infected health care workers have any knowledge of previous HBV infection or have symptoms at the time of detection. Similarly, more than 75% of cases are acquired from patients with previously undiagnosed disease.

In institutions for the mentally retarded, the risk of staff acquiring HBV infection is directly related to exposure to blood or blood products. Additional risks exist from bites, skin lesions, saliva, and other potentially infected secretions. As many as 30% of the residents in some institutions can be long-term carriers of HBsAg.

Ideally, health care workers should be vaccinated without screening when they are students or trainees. In other groups of health care workers with high rates (15% or more) of HBV marker positivity, it may be cost-effective to undertake serologic screening and vaccinate only those who are seronegative, although vaccinating persons who are already immune is not associated with increased risk for adverse reactions. Because seroresponsiveness to hepatitis B vaccine in adults is inversely related to age, it is recommended that after completing a three-dose series, the immunologic response should be determined by serologic testing for anti-HBs in persons age 30 years and older. In addition, testing for seroconversion may be advisable in younger adults at high occupational risk because as many as 5% of vaccine recipients ages 20 to 30 years will not develop protective levels of anti-HBs, even after revaccination. Persons who do not respond may wish to change their work assignments or responsibilities.

After acute needle-stick or mucosal exposure to blood, steps should be taken immediately to analyze the exposure incident and provide appropriate prophylaxis within 72 hours (Table 8.3). The HBsAg status of the patient and the anti-HBs status of the exposed, previously vaccinated health care worker should be determined if not already known. For the health care worker who is anti-HBs-positive, no further intervention is needed. If the patient is HBsAg positive and the health care worker is anti-HBs negative, hepatitis B immune globulin (HBIG) and hepatitis B vaccine should be given simultaneously at separate sites. Arrangements should be made for second and third doses of hepatitis B vaccine to be given 1 and 6 months later. If the patient who is the source of exposure is HBsAg negative, previously unvaccinated health care workers should be given a three-dose series of hepatitis B vaccine; HBIG is not required.

Influenza: Annual influenza immunization is strongly recommended for health care workers to reduce the likelihood of influenza transmission to patients. Vaccination also should reduce illness and absenteeism among health care workers during community outbreaks of influenza. Influenza vaccine should be given during the fall (ideally in October). Health care workers who have frequent contact with high-risk patients (for example, staff of intensive care units, geriatric units, nursing homes, and home health care agencies) should receive special priority. Immunization programs, especially those in hospitals, must be sure to reach personnel who work the evening and night shifts. If a community outbreak of influenza occurs, the vaccination status of all staff should be reviewed; those who have not been immunized should be.

Rubella: All health care workers who might transmit rubella to pregnant patients or to other health care workers should have documented serologic immunity or be vaccinated. Pregnant women should not receive rubella vaccine. Therefore, if they are not pregnant and are vaccinated, they should avoid becoming pregnant for the next 3 months. Serologic determination of rubella susceptibility before vaccination is not necessary; there is no increased risk for adverse reactions in vaccinating persons who are already immune. The combined measles, mumps, and rubella vaccine generally should be used.

Measles and Mumps: Recently, several outbreaks of measles were traced to health care settings. Measles vaccination is recommended for health care workers unless they were born before 1957 or have a record of physician-diagnosed measles or serologic evidence of immunity. Health care workers who have received a single measles immunization previously should be revaccinated at time of employment. Unvaccinated health care workers should receive two doses of vaccine, separated by no less than 1 month. Requiring at least one dose of vaccine also may be considered for health care workers born before 1957 who are likely to have occupational exposure to measles because 10% to 15% of such persons may not have had natural measles. During measles outbreaks in medical settings, all susceptible health care workers should be vaccinated. If exposed to measles, they should be relieved from direct patient contact from the 5th to the 21st day regardless of receipt of vaccine or immune globulin.

Although mumps is less contagious than measles or rubella, infection can be transmitted in health care facilities when community outbreaks of disease occur. Health care workers who do not have a documented history of mumps or mumps vaccination should be immunized, preferably with MMR.

Poliomyelitis: Because indigenous polio caused by wild viruses has not occurred in the United States since 1979, polio vaccine is not a high priority among health care workers. However, health care workers in close contact with patients who might be excreting polioviruses and laboratory workers who handle specimens from such patients should be immune to poliomyelitis. Persons who lack documentation of a completed primary series should complete the series with enhanced-potency inactivated polio vaccine. The inactivated vaccine is preferred because adults have a slightly increased risk for vaccine-associated paralytic poliomyelitis after receiving oral polio vaccination and because orally administered vaccine virus can be excreted for 30 days or more, thus possibly exposing immunocompromised patients to the risk for vaccine-associated paralytic poliomyelitis.

Tetanus-Diphtheria: Health care workers should keep current with recommendations for primary and booster immunizations with Td toxoids.

Essential Community Service Personnel

Persons who provide essential community services (policemen, firemen, school teachers, communications workers, and emergency medicine personnel, for example) should be considered for yearly influenza vaccination. Hepatitis B vaccine is recommended for emergency medicine personnel because of their frequent exposure to blood.

Day-Care Center Personnel

Because of their unique and intense exposure to young children, day-care center personnel should be fully protected against measles, mumps, and rubella. In addition, day-care center personnel should be considered for yearly influenza vaccination. *Haemophilus influenzae* type b vaccine is not needed because adults do not usually sustain disease. If an outbreak of hepatitis A occurs, day-care center personnel should be given immune globulin. When hepatitis A vaccine becomes available, susceptible day-care personnel will be among those targeted to receive it.

Laboratory Personnel

Laboratory personnel in most hospitals and private diagnostic laboratories who handle clinical specimens, especially blood, are at increased risk for acquiring hepatitis B and should be given pre-exposure prophylaxis with hepatitis B vaccine. They are not at high risk for other vaccine-preventable infections.

Personnel who work in specialized research and diagnostic laboratories may need additional vaccines—typhoid vaccine, for instance. Those involved with testing or isolating rabies virus should receive pre-exposure prophylaxis with rabies vaccine. Those working with *Francisella tularensis* or tularemia-infected animals should be considered for immunization with the live attenuated tularemia vaccine. Anthrax vaccine is indicated for laboratory workers performing studies involving *Bacillus anthracis*. Smallpox vaccination is indicated only for laboratory workers involved with orthopox viruses or with the production and testing of smallpox vaccine.

Veterinarians, Animal Handlers, Rural Workers, and Other Field Personnel

Because of their potential exposure to rabies, veterinarians and animal handlers should receive pre-exposure prophylaxis with rabies vaccine. Pre-exposure vaccination does not eliminate the need for additional post-exposure doses of rabies vaccine (Table 8.14). Persons whose risk for exposure is continuous should receive booster doses of rabies vaccine every 2 years or be tested for rabies antibody every 2 years and given booster doses if the titer level is less than that considered protective. Veterinarians and other persons who work in western and southwestern areas of the United States and who have regular field exposure to potentially plague-infected wild rodents, rabbits, and their fleas should be immunized with plague vaccine.

Persons who work in rural areas or who have extensive field exposure should be evaluated individually for their risks for several vaccine-preventable diseases. Forest rangers, laboratory animal handlers, and others likely to be exposed to potentially rabid dogs, cats, skunks, raccoons, bats, or other animals that might have rabies should receive pre-exposure prophylaxis as above. Anthrax is rarely seen in the United States. Anthrax vaccine is recommended only for persons whose occupations require frequent contact with imported animal products and for those who perform laboratory studies involving *B. anthracis*. The vaccine is available from the Biologic Products Program of the Michigan Department of Public Health.

Sanitation and Sewage Workers

Despite concern regarding disease transmission, sanitation and sewage workers do not appear to be at greater risk for hepatitis B or polio than the general population and do not require hepatitis B vaccine or a polio vaccine booster. Routine use of other immunizing agents such as typhoid vaccine or immune globulins also is not recommended. Vaccinations generally recommended for adults (for example, Td toxoids) should be given if indicated.

Immigrants and Refugees

The large influx of immigrants and refugees from southeast Asia and Latin America in recent years has increased physician awareness of the special infectious disease problems of developing countries. Risks have been particularly high for tuberculosis, hepatitis B, malaria, and gastrointestinal parasitic diseases. These diseases are often detected by clinical screening before arrival in this country. With the exception of hepatitis B and tuberculosis, the infectious diseases common to these groups have little potential for spread to resident populations in the United States.

An immunization program for recent immigrants and refugees should begin with a careful history, with the assistance of an interpreter if necessary. Immunization practices in some countries include the use of Bacille Calmette-Guérin vaccine, inactivated polio vaccine, and other vaccines not often or no longer given in the United States. Immunizations for refugees and immigrants are indicated primarily to protect them from diseases to which they remain susceptible. An equally important goal is to prevent the transmission of disease, especially hepatitis B, from parents and other household members to children.

Routine Vaccinations: It is prudent to assume that the vaccines routinely given to children in the United States have not been given to immigrants and refugees unless there is proof otherwise. The immunization history should establish whether a primary series of tetanus and diphtheria toxoids has been given. Most immigrants and refugees from developing countries have experienced natural infection with measles, mumps, and rubella viruses (if they have not received MMR), but some may still be susceptible. It is reasonable and safe to administer MMR to all except pregnant women. Many adults will be naturally immune to poliovirus infections. Because polio is no longer a threat in the United States, polio immunization is not a high priority for immigrants.

Hepatitis B: Hepatitis B is endemic in many developing countries, especially those in east Asia and sub-Saharan Africa. In persons from the Pacific Islands and in Alaskan Eskimos, the prevalence of hepatitis B carriers can be as high as 15%. In many countries, chronic hepatitis B is the primary cause of hepatocellular carcinoma. Screening immigrants and refugees for HBsAg is often cost-effective. Susceptible family members and sexual partners of HBV carriers are at risk for HBV infection and should be vaccinated (Table 8.2). Screening is especially important in women of childbearing age. Approximately 70% to 90% of infected infants will become long-term HBV carriers. Immediate postpartum administration of HBIG and hepatitis B vaccine (within 7 days) should be given to all infants born to mothers carrying HBV, regardless of whether the mother is e-antigen positive. This regimen is 90% to 95% effective in preventing HBV transmission from infected mothers to their newborn infants.

Tuberculosis: Mycobacterial infections affect as many as 50% to 70% of immigrants and refugees, as indicated by positive tuberculin reactions. A positive purified protein derivative skin test may reflect previous infection with either *Mycobacterium tuberculosis* or atypical mycobacteria, or it may indicate earlier Bacille Calmette-Guérin vaccination. However, a purified protein derivative reaction greater than 10 mm in induration should be interpreted as reflecting possible *M. tuberculosis* infection until proved otherwise. Prophylactic or therapeutic antituberculosis treatment should be considered.

Armed Forces Personnel

Former or current members of the U.S. Armed Forces, including the Coast Guard, and their dependents who may be on overseas assignments, will almost always have received their primary and required booster vaccinations. Veterans or active-duty Armed Forces personnel can be assumed to have been vaccinated at the time of induction into service. All military recruits (both enlisted men and officers) are given Td toxoids and oral polio, measles, rubella, and influenza vaccines. Before traveling to other countries, Armed Forces personnel may also be given hepatitis B, typhoid, cholera, plague, and meningococcal vaccines, among others. Some military personnel may still receive smallpox vaccine.

Risk Behaviors

Homosexual and Bisexual Men

Homosexual and bisexual men are at increased risk for HBV infection and should be vaccinated as soon as possible after becoming homosexually active. Without such protection, they have a 10% to 30% risk for acquiring HBV infection each year. Because a significant proportion of these men will already be infected, serologic screening is probably cost-effective. Hepatitis B vaccination is highly protective in otherwise healthy homosexual or bisexual men. However, in those who test positive for the human immunodeficiency virus, only 50% to 70% develop protective levels of antibody after hepatitis B vaccination. Despite widespread recognition of their susceptibility to hepatitis B, only a small minority of homosexual or bisexual men have received hepatitis B vaccine.

Injecting Drug Users

Approximately 50% to 80% of injecting drug users have serologic evidence of previous HBV infection. Prevaccination screening of these persons is probably cost-effective. In addition, special attention should be given to maintaining tetanus immunity in injecting drug users.

Prostitutes and Persons with Multiple Sexual Partners or Sexually Transmitted Diseases

Prostitutes and persons with multiple sexual partners or recently acquired sexually transmitted diseases are at increased risk for HBV infections, often as a result of concurrent intravenous drug use. Serologic screening and hepatitis B vaccination of susceptible persons is recommended.

5.

Immunizations for Accidental or Unavoidable Exposure

Wounds and Tetanus Prophylaxis

Primary immunization with tetanus toxoid provides 10 or more years of protection in all recipients. After a primary immunization series is complete, patients who suffer wounds that are severe or contaminated should receive booster doses if tetanus toxoid has not been given within the preceding 5 years. For lesser wounds, the tetanus and diphtheria (Td) booster interval is 10 years. Protective levels of circulating antitoxin develop rapidly in persons who have previously received at least two doses of tetanus toxoid. Table 5.1 provides a guide to tetanus prophylaxis in wound management.

Combined Td toxoid is preferred to tetanus toxoid alone for active tetanus immunization in managing wounds because it also enhances diphtheria protection among adults. Human tetanus immune globulin is used if passive immunization is needed. The recommended dose of tetanus immune globulin is 250 units administered intramuscularly. When tetanus toxoid and tetanus immune globulin are given concurrently, adsorbed rather than fluid tetanus toxoid should be given, and separate syringes and separate sites of injection should be used to prevent tetanus immune globulin from inactivating the tetanus toxoid.

Needle Stick/Sharps Injuries in Health Care Settings

In addition to local wound care, the major treatment decisions pertain to the use of hepatitis B vaccine and hepatitis B immune globulin (Table 8.3) and the use of chemoprophylaxis for infection with the human immunodeficiency virus. Data are insufficient to make recommendations for use of immune globulin to prevent hepatitis C.

Animal Bites and Rabies

Each possible rabies exposure should be evaluated individually. In the United States, risk factors to consider in determining the need for

TABLE 5.1. Summary Guide to Tetanus Prophylaxis* in Routine Wound Management, United States

	Clean, Minor Wounds		All Other Wounds[†]	
	Td[‡]	TIG[§]	Td	TIG
Uncertain or < 3	Yes	No	Yes	Yes
3 or more[‖]	No[¶]	No	No[**]	No

* Refer also to text on specific vaccines or toxoids for contraindications, precautions, dosages, side effects, adverse reactions, and special considerations. Important details are in the text and in the ACIP recommendations on diphtheria, tetanus, and pertussis (DTP) (MMWR. 1991; 40[RR-10]).

† Such as, but not limited to wounds contaminated with dirt, feces, and saliva; puncture wounds; avulsions; and wounds resulting from missiles, crushing, burns, and frostbite.

‡ Td = Tetanus and diphtheria toxoids, adsorbed (for adult use). For children 7 years old, DTP (DT, if pertussis vaccine is contraindicated) is preferred to tetanus toxoid alone. For persons 7 years old, Td is preferred to tetanus toxoid alone.

§ TIG = Tetanus immune globulin.

‖ If only three doses of fluid toxoid have been received, a fourth dose of toxoid, preferably an adsorbed toxoid, should be given.

¶ Yes. >10 years since last dose.

** Yes. >5 years since last dose. (More frequent boosters are not needed and can accentuate side effects.)

Source: Centers for Disease Control. Update on adult immunization. MMWR. 1991;40 (RR-12):1–94.

antirabies treatment include the species of the animal, circumstances of the biting incident, type of exposure, and geographic region in which the incident occurred.

Some animals are more likely than others to be infected with rabies virus. Carnivorous wild animals (especially skunks, raccoons, foxes, coyotes, and bobcats), bats, and woodchucks are the animals most commonly infected. Even if exposure to one of these animals was provoked, postexposure prophylaxis (Table 8.13) should be initiated promptly unless the animal can be immediately tested and shown not to be rabid. The likelihood that a domestic dog or cat is infected with rabies virus varies from region to region; thus, the need for postexposure prophylaxis also varies. Rodents such as squirrels, hamsters, guinea pigs, gerbils, chipmunks, rats, mice, and lagomorphs (rabbits and hares) are rarely found to be infected and have not been known to cause human rabies in the United States; therefore, their bites do not routinely require antirabies prophylaxis.

Knowledge of the circumstances of the biting incident is useful in making management decisions. An unprovoked attack is more likely than a provoked attack to indicate that the animal is rabid. Bites inflicted when a person was attempting to feed or handle an apparently healthy animal should generally be regarded as provoked.

The type, nature, and extent of exposure should help determine the likelihood that rabies infection will result from exposure. Rabies is transmitted by introducing the virus into open skin cuts or wounds or through mucous membranes. A bite exposure includes any penetration of the skin by teeth. A nonbite exposure includes scratches, abrasions, and open wounds or contact with mucous membranes that are contaminated with saliva or other infectious material (such as brain tissue) from a rabid or a potentially rabid animal. Casual contact such as petting does not constitute an exposure and is not an indication for prophylaxis. Local or state public health officials should be consulted if questions arise about the need for rabies prophylaxis.

Postexposure prophylaxis begins with immediate cleansing of the wound with soap and water. A guide to postexposure prophylaxis with rabies vaccine and human rabies immune globulin is given in Table 8.14. For postexposure immunization, rabies vaccine should be administered intramuscularly (not intradermally). The deltoid area is the preferred site; the buttock should be avoided. Human rabies immune globulin is used for passive prophylaxis. Rabies vaccine and human rabies immune globulin should be administered in separate syringes at separate anatomic sites.

Snake Bites

Most poisonous snake bites in the United States are inflicted by pit vipers (crotalid snakes), including all rattlesnakes, cottonmouths, and copperheads. A polyvalent antivenin for pit vipers is produced by Wyeth-Ayerst Laboratories (Philadelphia, Pennsylvania) and is called Antivenin (*Crotalidae*), polyvalent. A separate antivenin directed at eastern coral snake venom, called Antivenin (*Micrurus fulvius*), is also available from Wyeth-Ayerst Laboratories. These antivenins are hyperimmune horse serum preparations. Their use is associated with an immediate risk for anaphylaxis and a delayed risk for serum sickness.

The need for antivenin and the required dose are determined by the severity of the bite and subsequent envenomation, as well as by the type of snake involved. For example, a penetrating bite by a Mojave rattlesnake or an eastern coral snake is an indication for early and aggressive use of the appropriate antivenin. For bites by pit vipers other than the Mojave rattlesnake, the severity of envenomation and the patient's signs and symptoms determine the dose of antivenin to be used.

Whenever possible, antivenin therapy should be instituted within the first 4 hours after the bite. For rattlesnake bites with minimal envenomation, 3 to 4 vials of antivenin (30 to 40 mL reconstituted) should suffice.

Moderate or severe bites can require 5 to 15 or more vials. The antivenin should be given intravenously in most instances, but only after skin testing to determine if the patient is allergic to horse serum. The occurrence of serum sickness as a late complication of antivenin therapy is dose dependent; it can be expected in almost all patients who receive more than 7 vials (70 mL) of antivenin. Prophylactic tetanus vaccination should be given if indicated.

Spider Bites

Almost all spiders are venomous, but in the United States severe illness and death are associated with the bites of only two species, the black widow (*Latrodectus mactans*) and the brown recluse (*Loxosceles reclusa*). Deaths from spider bites are rare, and approximately 95% are attributed to the black widow spider.

An antivenin directed against black widow spider venom is produced by Merck, Sharp & Dohme (West Point, Pennsylvania) and is called Black Widow Spider Species antivenin. The product is of equine origin; consequently, its use is associated with an immediate risk for anaphylaxis and a delayed risk for serum sickness. No antivenin directed at brown recluse spider venom is available.

For most black widow spider bites, treatment is symptomatic and supportive. The need for antivenin and the dose required are generally dictated by the severity of the bite and the progression of the patient's symptoms. Antivenin therapy is recommended for patients with hypertensive cardiovascular disease and for those younger than 16 or older than 60 years. The dose is one vial (2.5 mL) given intravenously in saline after skin testing to determine if the patient is allergic to horse serum. Antivenin therapy for black widow spider bites should not be regarded as essential; most bites can be treated satisfactorily by supportive measures alone. When antivenin is used, the amount required is substantially less than that used for snake bites, so serum sickness is less likely to occur. Tetanus prophylaxis should be given if indicated.

Immunizations for Communicable Disease Exposure

Meningococcal Infections

Vaccination with quadrivalent A, C, Y, and W-135 meningococcal polysaccharide vaccine should be considered when an outbreak of meningococcal infection caused by a vaccine serogroup organism occurs in a closed or semiclosed population. Vaccination may serve as an adjunct to antimicrobial chemoprophylaxis with rifampin, ciprofloxacin, or ceftriaxone (or a sulfonamide if the organism is sulfonamide-susceptible) for close individual or family contacts of persons with meningococcal disease. Because as many as one half of secondary cases of meningococcal disease occur more than 5 days after the primary infection, vaccination may be beneficial in a closed or semiclosed setting.

Hepatitis A

Immune globulin is recommended for postexposure prophylaxis for close household and sexual contacts of persons with hepatitis A; staff and attendees of day-care centers and members of households with diapered children who attend day-care centers in which hepatitis A transmission is occurring; selected staff and patients of custodial institutions in which hepatitis A is occurring; and coworkers of persons with hepatitis A who handle food. A single dose of immune globulin (0.02 mL/kg) should be given intramuscularly as soon as possible after exposure. Immune globulin prophylaxis given more than 2 weeks after exposure is unlikely to be beneficial and is not indicated. Immune globulin is not recommended for casual contacts of persons with hepatitis A (for example, coworkers in an office setting or school contacts), nor is it generally recommended for patrons of a restaurant in which hepatitis A occurred in a person who handled food. Its use is recommended, however, for control of food-borne outbreaks. It is anticipated that hepatitis A vaccine (soon to be licensed) will replace immune globulin for prevention of hepatitis A in most pre-exposure situations, but immune globulin will likely remain the postexposure treatment of choice.

Hepatitis B

Postexposure prophylaxis for hepatitis B virus infection should be considered for persons having accidental percutaneous or mucosal exposure to blood or body fluids known or suspected to contain hepatitis B surface antigen (HBsAg), and for persons having intimate or sexual exposure to someone who is HBsAg positive. Specific guidelines for postexposure prophylaxis with hepatitis B immune globulin (HBIG) and hepatitis B vaccine are given in Table 8.3. Because health care workers who have accidental percutaneous or mucosal exposures are candidates for hepatitis B vaccine, hepatitis B vaccine and HBIG should be administered simultaneously; this provides long-term and short-term protection. Postexposure prophylaxis is also indicated for persons sexually exposed to HBsAg-positive persons if HBIG and the first dose of vaccine can be given within 14 days of exposure or if sexual contact with the infected person will continue. For exposed persons who have previously received pre-exposure prophylaxis with one or more doses of hepatitis B vaccine, the decision to provide additional postexposure prophylaxis should be based on the source of exposure and on the anti-hepatitis B antigen status of the vaccinated person (Table 8.3).

Hepatitis C

No firm recommendation can be made for postexposure prophylaxis for hepatitis C. Results of studies of postexposure prophylaxis for hepatitis C are equivocal. For persons with percutaneous exposure to blood from a patient with parenterally transmitted non-A, non-B hepatitis, some authorities believe it is reasonable to administer immune globulin (0.06 mg/kg) as soon as possible after exposure. There is evidence that hepatitis C virus infection does not elicit protective immunity in chimpanzees, suggesting that there may be problems in efforts to prevent this disease by passive or active immunization.

Varicella Zoster

Postexposure prophylaxis with varicella zoster immune globulin is indicated for immunocompromised persons who are thought to be susceptible to varicella and have been closely exposed to someone with active varicella or zoster lesions (Table 8.6). Susceptible pregnant women and infants born to mothers in whom varicella develops within 5 days or before 48 hours after delivery also should receive varicella zoster immune globulin.

Measles

Nonimmune contacts of patients with active measles should receive immune globulin (Table 8.6).

Botulism

Botulinus antitoxin (trivalent, types A, B, and E) is available for the treatment and prevention of botulism through the Centers for Disease Control and Prevention. The efficacy of botulinus antitoxin has not been established clearly but is believed to be beneficial, particularly if given early in the course of the disease. The antitoxin does not reverse the activity of toxin already bound to nerve endings but does appear to neutralize circulating unbound toxin.

This antitoxin is of equine origin and the probability of serum sickness, seen in about 10% of treated patients, is dose-related. The dosage recommendations from the Centers for Disease Control and Prevention should be followed closely.

6.

Immunizations for Immunocompromised Adults

The acquired immunodeficiency syndrome has focused attention on the prevention of infections in patients with altered host defenses. Advances in transplantation and cancer chemotherapy and development of aggressive immunosuppressive therapy for a variety of conditions have increased the life spans of patients with end-stage heart, liver, and kidney diseases, carcinomas, and autoimmune diseases. The major threat to the health of these patients is no longer their primary diseases but rather the infectious disease complications related to their therapies.

In preventing infection in patients with human immunodeficiency virus (HIV) infection and in those with other congenital and acquired defects in host defenses, four general principles should be remembered. First, prevention of infection is far better than treatment, particularly for patients with severe defects in host defenses. Second, the need for preventive efforts is determined by the circumstances of the exposure to infection for each patient. Third, the likelihood of both acquiring and preventing infection is directly related to the patient's net state of immunosuppression and the severity of the disease. Fourth, vaccine efficacy is often diminished in immunocompromised patients. Recognize that immunization recommendations for these patients are rarely based on rigorous clinical trials. Rather, in most instances recommendations represent clinical logic based on the incidence and severity of the disease and the safety of the vaccine.

Formerly, the study of immunodeficiency disorders emphasized the rare patient with an isolated, usually congenital, defect in host defense (for example, X-linked agammaglobulinemia and the DiGeorge syndrome). Now, however, most immunocompromised adults have acquired conditions with complex abnormalities of host defense. Rather than relating the risk for infection and the need for preventive strategies to one particular characteristic, such as a disease or its therapy, the concept of net state of immunosuppression has emerged. The net state of immunosuppression is determined by the interaction of a number of variables, including 1) the underlying disease and age; 2) the dose and duration of the immunosuppressive therapy; 3) humoral and cellular host defenses; 4) the integrity of the skin and mucosal surfaces of the body; 5) metabolic factors such as malnutrition, uremia, hyperglycemia, and, probably, hepatic dysfunction; 6) abnormalities of the reticuloendothelial system, most notably the absence of splenic function; and 7) the presence or absence of immunomodulating infections such as those caused by HIV, cytomegalovirus, and, probably, hepatitis viruses and Epstein-Barr virus. Although the net state of immunosuppression determines the risk for infection and the need for prevention, it also influences the effectiveness and safety of preventive immunologic interventions.

Tables 6.1 to 6.3 summarize the recommended indications, cautions, and conditions for vaccines and immunoglobulins given to immunocompromised patients.

HIV Infection and the Acquired Immunodeficiency Syndrome

The immune compromise resulting from HIV infection is multifactorial. First, the critically important helper-inducer subset of T lymphocytes (the CD4 lymphocytes) is depleted and infection of an important subset of monocytes and macrophages occurs. These events produce defects in cell-mediated immunity that permit the occurrence of a broad array of opportunistic infections, primarily those caused by intracellular microbial parasites. Two of these infections, measles and varicella, can be prevented with active or passive immunization.

Measles virus can cause disseminated, fatal disease in susceptible HIV-infected persons. Limited studies with measles vaccine in symptomatic or asymptomatic HIV-infected patients have not found serious or unusual side effects. Measles vaccine (preferably given as measles, mumps, and rubella [MMR] vaccine) is recommended in the absence of a physician-documented diagnosis of measles, serologic evidence of immunity, or a history of receipt of two doses at least 1 month apart.

In symptomatic HIV-infected patients (that is, those with CD4 counts less than $200/mm^3$) exposed to measles, immune globulin should be given regardless of previous immune status because the vaccine may not be effective in such patients. If given, measles vaccine is more likely to be effective when given within 3 days of exposure. The dose of immune globulin is 0.5 mL/kg (15 mL maximum) intramuscularly (which is twice the recommended dose). Immune globulin should be given within 6 days of exposure. Immune globulin may not be necessary in patients receiving 100 to 400 mg/kg of intravenous immune globulin regularly with the last dose having been given within 3 weeks of exposure to measles.

TABLE 6.1. Summary of ACIP Recommendations on Immunization of Immunocompromised Adults

Vaccine	Routine (Not Immuno-compromised)	HIV Infection/AIDS	Severely Immuno-compromised (non-HIV related)*	After Solid Organ Transplant or Chronic Immunosuppressive Therapy	Asplenia	Renal Failure	Diabetes	Alcoholism and Alcoholic Cirrhosis
Td	Recommended	Recommended	Recommended	Recommended	Recommended	Recommended	Recommended	Recommended
MMR(MR/M/R)†	Use if indicated	Recommended/considered‡	Contraindicated	Contraindicated	Use if indicated	Use if indicated	Use if indicated	Use if indicated
Hepatitis B	Use if indicated	Use if indicated	Use if indicated	Use if indicated	Use if indicated	Recommended§	Use if indicated	Use if indicated
Hib	Not recommended	Considered‖	Recommended	Recommended	Recommended	Use if indicated	Use if indicated	Use if indicated
Pneumococcal	Recommended if ≥65 years	Recommended	Recommended	Recommended	Recommended	Recommended	Recommended	Recommended
Meningococcal	Use if indicated	Use if indicated	Use if indicated	Use if indicated	Recommended	Use if indicated	Use if indicated	Use if indicated
Influenza	Recommended if ≥65 years	Recommended	Recommended	Recommended	Recommended	Recommended	Recommended	Recommended

* Severe immunosuppression can be the result of congenital immunodeficiency, leukemia, lymphoma, generalized malignancy, or therapy with alkylating agents, antimetabolites, radiation, or large amounts of corticosteroids.

† MMR = measles-mumps-rubella vaccine; M = measles only; M/R = measles and rubella only.

‡ See discussion of MMR in section on human immunodeficiency virus (HIV) and the acquired immunodeficiency syndrome (AIDS).

§ Patients with renal failure receiving dialysis should have their anti-Hbs response tested after vaccination, and those who do not respond should be revaccinated.

‖ *See* discussion of HIV.

Source: Modified from Centers for Disease Control and Prevention. Recommendations of the Advisory Committee on Immunization Practices: use of vaccines and immunoglobulins in persons with altered immunocompetence. MMWR 1993;42(RR-5):1–18.

Disseminated primary varicella zoster virus infection can be a rapidly progressive, fatal illness in patients with HIV. Treatment with varicella zoster immune globulin after exposure to varicella zoster virus is indicated for HIV-infected patients who have a negative varicella history or who lack antibodies to varicella zoster virus. It is important to recognize that varicella zoster immune globlin may only modify the clinical illness and not provide complete protection. Thus, in the HIV-infected patient who has received varicella zoster immune globulin prophylaxis, the possibility of disseminated varicella zoster virus infection must be considered if within the next month the patient has fever and abdominal or central nervous system complaints even without rash. In such a case, intravenous acyclovir therapy may be life-saving.

In addition to the primary defect in cell-mediated immunity, HIV-infected patients may have profound defects in humoral immunity. These defects are not due to direct infection of B lymphocytes, but rather to their polyclonal activation, which results in several abnormalities, the most important of which is a decreased antibody response (particularly IgM) to primary immunizations. These defects result in an increased risk for infection by *Streptococcus pneumoniae* and *Haemophilus influenzae* type b, encapsulated bacteria that require antibody for effective opsonization. Therefore, pneumococcal vaccine is recommended, and *H. influenzae* type b conjugate vaccine should be considered for HIV-infected patients, even though their efficacies may be less than expected in the general population.

It has not been shown that HIV-infected adults are at increased risk for death as a result of influenza. Nevertheless, it is reasonable to vaccinate these patients annually even though the antibody response to influenza vaccine may be suboptimal. Regardless of influenza vaccination status, HIV-infected patients in whom influenza-like illness develops during community outbreaks of type A influenza are candidates for rimantadine/amantadine treatment.

Bacille Calmette-Guérin vaccine should be avoided in HIV-infected persons because of reported complications. Other live attenuated vaccines that should be avoided in HIV-infected persons and others who are severely immunocompromised are the Ty2la typhoid vaccine, oral polio vaccine, yellow fever vaccine, and vaccinia. Killed vaccine alternatives are available for typhoid and polio.

When healthy household members are immunized against polio, inactive polio vaccine should be given to avoid spread of live oral polio virus to an immunocompromised patient.

TABLE 6.2. Summary of ACIP Recommendations on Nonroutine Immunization of Immunocompromised Persons*

Vaccine	Not Immuno-compromised	HIV Infection/AIDS	Severely Immuno-compromised (Non-HIV Related)[†]	After Solid Organ Transplant or Chronic Immunosuppressive Therapy	Asplenia, Renal Failure, Diabetes, Alcoholism, and Alcoholic Cirrhosis
Live vaccines					
BCG	Use if indicated	Contraindicated	Contraindicated	Contraindicated	Use if indicated
OPV	Use if indicated	Contraindicated	Contraindicated	Contraindicated	Use if indicated
Vaccinia	Use if indicated	Contraindicated	Contraindicated	Contraindicated	Use if indicated
Typhoid, Ty21a	Use if indicated	Contraindicated	Contraindicated	Contraindicated	Use if indicated
Yellow fever[‡]	Use if indicated	Contraindicated	Contraindicated	Contraindicated	Use if indicated
Killed or inactivated vaccines					
IPV	Use if indicated	Use if indicated	Use if indicated	Use if indicated	Use if indicated
Cholera	Use if indicated	Use if indicated	Use if indicated	Use if indicated	Use if indicated
Plague	Use if indicated	Use if indicated	Use if indicated	Use if indicated	Use if indicated
Typhoid, inactivated	Use if indicated	Use if indicated	Use if indicated	Use if indicated	Use if indicated
Rabies	Use if indicated	Use if indicated	Use if indicated	Use if indicated	Use if indicated
Anthrax	Use if indicated	Use if indicated	Use if indicated	Use if indicated	Use if indicated

* BCG = Bacille Calmette-Guérin; OPV = oral polio vaccine; IPV = inactivated polio vaccine; HIV = human immunodeficiency virus; AIDS = acquired immunodeficiency syndrome.

[†] Severe immunosuppression also can be the result of congenital immunodeficiency, leukemia, lymphoma, aplastic anemia, generalized malignancy, or therapy with alkylating agents, antimetabolites, radiation, or large amounts of corticosteroids.

[‡] Yellow fever vaccine should be considered for patients when exposure to yellow fever cannot be avoided (*see* text).

Source: Modified from Centers for Disease Control and Prevention. Recommendations of the Advisory Committee on Immunization Practices: use of vaccines and immunoglobulins in persons with altered immunocompetence. MMWR 1993;42 (RR-5): 1–18.

Splenic Disorders

Patients with surgical or functional asplenia (for example, sickle cell disease) have reduced clearance of encapsulated bacteria from the bloodstream, resulting in an increased risk for overwhelming infection, caused most often by *S. pneumoniae* and *H. influenzae* type b. The individual lifetime risk for such infections may approach 5% if splenectomy is done during a staging procedure for hematologic malignancy or for the treatment of hemolytic anemia or thalassemia. The risk is considerably less for patients who have splenectomy after trauma because splenic rests remain in the peritoneum when the spleen is ruptured. Pneumococcal vaccine is indicated for all asplenic persons. If possible, vaccination should be given at least 2 weeks before elective splenectomy to ensure a maximum antibody response. Persons previously given 14-valent vaccine should be reimmunized with 23-valent vaccine (licensed in 1983), and all asplenic persons should be revaccinated if more than 6 years has elapsed since initial vaccination. *Haemophilus influenzae* type b conjugate vaccine and meningococcal vaccine should also be considered for asplenic persons. In addition, the importance of antimalarial prophylaxis must be emphasized for those planning foreign travel to areas where malaria occurs.

Diabetes Mellitus

Results of several in-vitro tests of host defense function are known to be abnormal in patients with diabetes. Because patients with long-standing diabetes mellitus often also have cardiovascular, renal, and other end-organ dysfunction, pneumococcal and influenza vaccines are indicated.

Renal Failure

Patients with renal failure have an increased risk for infection with a variety of pathogens, especially pneumococcus. The nephrotic syndrome is the renal disease most clearly associated with an increased risk for pneumococcal infection. The efficacy of pneumococcal vaccine in patients with renal failure may be lower compared with that in healthy persons, and the antibody levels have been shown to decrease more rapidly. Consequently, patients with renal failure, including those receiving dialysis and those with the nephrotic syndrome, should receive repeated vaccination every 3 to 5 years. Immunization should be given early in the course of progressive renal disease, especially if kidney transplant and chronic immunosuppressive therapy are contemplated.

TABLE 6.3. Summary of ACIP Recommendations on Use of Immune Globulins in Immunocompromised Persons*

Immune Globulin	Not Immunocompromised	HIV Infected	Severely Immunocompromised[†]
IG	Recommended for infants and susceptible adults exposed to measles	Recommended for symptomatic patients exposed to measles regardless of immunization status Recommended for persons with exposure to hepatitis A or who will travel to HAV-endemic areas	Recommended for patients exposed to measles regardless of immunization status
VZIG	May be used for exposed susceptible adults and exposed susceptible pregnant women, and infants <28 days	Recommended for susceptible infants and adults after significant exposure to V-Z	Recommended for adults after significant exposure to V-Z
TIG	Recommended for those with serious wounds and <3 doses of tetanus toxoid	Same as for non-immunocompromised	Same as for nonimmuno-compromised
HBIG	Recommended for prophylaxis in susceptible persons with percutaneous, sexual, or mucosal exposure to HBV	Same as for non-immunocompromised	Same as for nonimmuno-compromised
HRIG	Recommended for postexposure prophylaxis of persons not previously vaccinated against rabies	Same as for non-immunocompromised	Same as for nonimmuno-compromised

* IG = immune globulin; HIV = human immunodeficiency virus; VZIG = varicella zoster IG; TIG = tetanus IG; HBIG = hepatitis B IG; HRIG = human rabies IG; V-Z = varicella zoster; HAV = hepatitis A virus; HBV = hepatitis B virus.

[†] Severe immunosuppression also can be the result of congenital immunodeficiency, leukemia, lymphoma, aplastic anemia, generalized malignancy or therapy with alkylating agents, antimetabolites, radiation, or large amounts of corticosteroids.

[‡] *See* Chapter 8, Immune Globulin for a discussion of issues to be considered before using VZIG.

Source: Modified from Centers for Disease Control and Prevention. Recommendations of the Advisory Committee on Immunization Practices: use of vaccines and immunoglobulins in persons with altered immunocompetence. MMWR 1993;42 (RR-5): 1–18.

Hepatitis B vaccine is indicated for patients whose renal disease is likely to lead to dialysis or kidney transplantation. Such patients have an increased risk for hepatitis B because of their need for blood products and hemodialysis. Unfortunately, after end-stage renal disease develops, hepatitis B vaccination is less effective than it is in the general population, as measured by seroconversion rates, antibody titers, and long-term antibody persistence. Higher doses of the vaccine are available and should be used for patients receiving hemodialysis or persons who are immunosuppressed. In addition, periodic booster doses are usually necessary after successful immunization, with their timing determined by serologic testing at 6- to 12-month intervals.

Patients with chronic renal failure should receive yearly influenza immunization. Because the efficacy of influenza vaccine may be less in these patients than in healthy persons, rimantadine prophylaxis or treatment or both may be considered during periods of increased type A influenza activity in the community. Rimantadine, which is metabolized in the liver, is preferred to amantadine (which is excreted by the kidneys) in patients with renal failure.

Alcoholism and Cirrhosis

Patients with alcoholism and alcoholic liver disease have an increased incidence of infections, especially tuberculosis and pneumonia. The defects in host defense in such patients are many, although the clinical significance of any one defect as measured in the laboratory is often uncertain. Malnutrition and a decreased ability to protect the airway are important factors. In addition, leukopenia, decreased complement activity, chemotactic defects, and impaired cell-mediated immunity occur in many of these patients. In those with cirrhosis, portosystemic shunting can diminish the clearance of bacteria, increasing the severity of infection. Patients who are alcoholics or have alcoholic liver disease should be immunized with pneumococcal and influenza vaccines.

Hepatitis B virus infections may play a role in development of chronic active hepatitis and hepatocellular carcinoma in alcoholic patients.

Organ Transplantation and Long-Term Corticosteroid, Azathioprine, Cyclophosphamide, or Cyclosporine Therapy

Defects in cell-mediated immunity develop in organ transplant patients who receive long-term immunosuppressive therapy. Similar treatment is also given to patients with collagen-vascular diseases, chronic active hepatitis, inflammatory bowel disease, and other inflammatory conditions. Immunization strategies for these patients are complicated by two problems. First, vaccines may be relatively ineffective. For example, fewer than 20% of renal transplant recipients receiving immunosuppressive therapy who are given hepatitis B vaccine may have protective levels of antibody 12 months later. Pneumococcal and influenza vaccines may also be less effective than in healthy persons. Second, vaccination might trigger a nonspecific immunologic response, resulting in allograft rejection or increased auto-immune activity. There is no evidence that this occurs after hepatitis B, influenza, or pneumococcal vaccination. However, anecdotal reports of renal allograft injury after administration of tetanus toxoid exist, and some transplant centers prefer to use tetanus immune globulin rather than booster doses of tetanus toxoid to manage tetanus-prone wounds. For these reasons, primary immunizations should be administered before immunosuppressive therapy is begun or when such therapy is at its lowest level. If this is not possible, postexposure protection with immune globulin preparations and antimicrobial or antiviral chemoprophylaxis or chemotherapy should be considered (*see* Chapter 5).

When healthy household members are immunized against polio, inactivated polio vaccine should be given to avoid spread of live oral polio virus to an immunocompromised patient.

Malignant Diseases

Patients with malignant diseases vary with respect to their risks for infection and their need for vaccines and immune globulin prophylaxis. Those with solid tumors (nonhematologic carcinomas) risk infection because of debility, anatomic compromise, and chemotherapy or radiation therapy. They should receive pneumococcal vaccine and yearly influenza immunization. Patients with hematologic carcinomas are considerably more immuno-compromised. Live attenuated virus vaccines such as MMR should be avoided except in those in remission who have received no chemotherapy for at least 3 months, but these patients should receive influenza and pneumococcal vaccines. Immunization should be timed carefully to avoid cycles of chemotherapy. If possible, vaccines should be administered before radiation therapy or splenectomy. This is especially important for patients with lymphoma in whom splenectomy is planned. The efficacy of influenza and pneumococcal vaccines in patients with chronic lymphocytic leukemia, B-cell lymphomas, and multiple myeloma may be limited. The effectiveness of replacement therapy with intravenous immune globulin in these patients is uncertain. Finally, patients with no previous experience with vari-cella zoster virus infection should receive varicella zoster immune globulin if they are exposed to this virus.

When healthy household members are immunized against polio, inac-tive polio vaccine should be given to avoid spread of live oral polio virus to immunocompromised patients.

Congenital and Acquired Immunodeficiency Diseases

Because of more effective medical care, many patients with congenital immunodeficiency disorders live to be adults. In general, vaccines are not effective in most of these patients. Live attenuated virus vaccines should be avoided, including oral polio vaccine, which can cause progressive menin-goencephalitis in immunoglobulin-deficient persons. Patients with X-linked agammaglobulinemia, X-linked immunodeficiency with hyper-IgM, and common variable hypogammaglobulinemia should receive replacement immune globulin therapy to maintain serum levels of IgG at 300 to 500 mg/dL. This can be done more easily and with less discomfort with the newer intravenous preparations than with intramuscular injections.

When healthy household members are immunized against polio, inac-tive polio vaccine should be given to avoid spread of live oral polio virus to immunocompromised patients.

Special consideration should be given to selective IgA deficiency, a con-dition affecting approximately 1 in every 700 persons. Because respirato-ry infections can be a frequent problem, these patients should be given pneu-mococcal and influenza vaccines. Immune globulin preparations should not be given. They will not correct IgA deficiency, and the trace amounts of IgA present can sensitize patients and lead to anaphylactic reactions.

Summary

From a practical standpoint, patients with immunocompromising dis-orders can be divided into three groups (Tables 6.1 to 6.3): 1) those with HIV infection; 2) those who have severe immunosuppression not due to HIV; and 3) those with other conditions that cause limited immune deficits such as asplenia, renal failure, diabetes, and alcoholism.

In general, killed vaccines can be given to patients in all three groups. Live virus vaccines are generally contraindicated in all patients in group 2, in some patients in group 1, and in none in group 3. Immunoglobulins are given to supplement vaccine-induced immunity in certain settings. Healthy persons such as family members or nursing personnel who have close contact with immunocompromised patients should not receive oral polio virus vaccine but may receive MMR. When polio vaccine is indicated, inactive polio vaccine should be used.

The effect of steroid therapy on the safety of live virus vaccines depends on dose and duration of treatment. Precise data are not available. In general, live virus vaccines can be used when corticosteroid therapy is short term (that is, for fewer than 2 weeks) or is administered topically by inhalation or by intra-articular, bursal, or tendon injection. A daily 20-mg prednisone regimen or equivalent doses of other corticosteroids can cause immunosuppression and raises concern about the safety of live virus vaccines. In addition, corticosteroid doses greater than physiologic doses (5 mg of prednisone) may reduce the immune response to vaccines. Patients who receive high doses of systemic steroids for 2 weeks or longer should not be vaccinated until 3 or more months after therapy is discontinued.

Future Directions

The increased number of immunocompromised patients at risk for acquiring life-threatening infection illustrates the importance of developing new approaches to preventing infection in this group. These approaches should include 1) the development and widespread use of simple, rapid serologic tests to determine immunity to such diseases as measles and varicella in immunocompromised persons; 2) the development of improved vaccines and specific hyperimmune globulin preparations; and 3) the development of new immune-modulating interventions such as safe and effective adjuvants that can be incorporated into vaccines and used in immunocompromised patients. A live attenuated varicella zoster virus vaccine will offer protection to susceptible adults. Development of a pneumococcal polysaccharide conjugate vaccine similar to *H. influenzae* type b conjugate vaccine may provide better protection for some immunocompromised patients. New approaches based on passive protection with specific hyperimmune globulin preparations appear to be promising. In the long term, however, the development of immune-modulating agents and adjuvants that improve responsiveness to active immunization is still an important goal.

7.

Immunizations and Other Preventive Measures for International Travel

More than 10 million Americans travel outside the United States annually. Most travelers have health-related questions that commonly fall into three categories: (1) What immunizations are indicated? (2) What health maintenance measures are necessary regarding food, drink, and other activities? and (3) What should I do if I get sick? Promotional materials for international travelers de-emphasize health problems and travel agents generally are not well informed about international health hazards.

An essential reference for physicians who advise travelers is the pamphlet *Health Information for International Travel*. It is published annually by the U.S. Public Health Service and can be obtained from the Centers for Disease Control and Prevention, Division of Quarantine, Atlanta, GA 30333, or from the Superintendent of Documents, U.S. Government Printing Office, Washington, DC 20402 (202-783-3238). The World Health Organization (WHO) publishes *Vaccination Certificate Requirements and Health Advice for International Travel*, which can be obtained from the WHO Regional Office for the Americas, 525 Twenty-third Street NW, Washington, DC 20037. Each book contains a compendium of vaccination certificate requirements for all countries, recommendations for immunization, prophylaxis for malaria and other diseases, and a useful set of health hints for the traveler. Both books are authoritative and easy to use. Some commercial publishers also have produced useful books on travel medicine. The Centers for Disease Control and Prevention maintains a Traveler's Hotline (404-332-4555) that provides touch-tone telephone access to the latest travel information.

Immunizations

The physician's advice to the traveler regarding immunizations is influenced by 1) the specific itinerary, 2) the entry or exit requirements for yellow fever or other vaccinations of countries visited, 3) the type of accommodations the traveler anticipates using, 4) the duration of travel, 5) the patient's status regarding routine immunizations, 6) the traveler's medical history, and 7) special requirements for Peace Corps personnel, missionaries, anthropologists, and others who anticipate living "close to the soil." This chapter summarizes indications for individual vaccines and immune globulins; more detailed discussions can be found in Chapter 8.

Routine Immunizations

When addressing the health concerns of travelers, the physician must review routinely recommended immunizations. These immunizations include pneumococcal and influenza vaccines for elderly and other high-risk persons, and completion of a primary series or a booster dose of combined tetanus-diphtheria toxoid.

Poliomyelitis: Travelers to areas where poliomyelitis is endemic or epidemic should have completed a primary series of polio vaccination. Because oral polio vaccine has rarely been associated with paralytic complications, enhanced-potency inactivated polio vaccine is preferred for primary immunization of previously unimmunized adults. For travelers who have completed a primary series, a one-time booster dose of either oral polio vaccine or enhanced-potency inactivated polio vaccine is advised. For patients who are immunocompromised, oral polio vaccine is contraindicated, and enhanced-potency inactivated polio vaccine should be used.

Measles, Mumps, and Rubella: Measles, mumps, and rubella are common diseases in developing countries. Susceptible travelers have become infected abroad and have been responsible for outbreaks of disease when they returned to the United States. Therefore, young adults who have not been vaccinated and have not contracted these diseases must be protected. Furthermore, one dose of measles, mumps, and rubella vaccine should be given to international travelers born after 1956 who have not previously received two doses and do not have other evidence of immunity.

Required Immunizations

Each country determines its own vaccination requirements for travelers. In recent years, the indications for required vaccines have become more narrowly defined. Vaccination against smallpox is no longer required for international travel and should not be given. In 1988, the World Health Organization eliminated its recommendation for cholera vaccination. Yellow fever vaccination is required only for travel to endemic areas, and meningococcal vaccine is required for entry into Saudi Arabia during the time of the annual pilgrimage to Mecca.

Yellow Fever: Yellow fever is endemic in equatorial Africa and in parts of South America. No cases have been reported among United States tourists in many years, and the risk among conventional travelers for developing yellow fever is small. Nevertheless, a number of countries require vaccination of all visitors, and others require it for travelers arriving from or proceeding to "infected areas." In the United States, yellow fever vaccine can be obtained only from designated public health approved centers. Because the vaccine contains the live 17D strain of yellow fever virus, patients who are immunocompromised and those who are hypersensitive to eggs should not be vaccinated. Pregnancy is a relative contraindication to vaccination, but for the pregnant women who *must* travel to areas where the risk for yellow fever is high, the benefit of vaccination may outweigh the theoretical risk to the fetus.

Some countries require an International Certificate of Vaccination for yellow fever for entry and exiting. The certificate is valid for a period from 10 days to 10 years after immunization. The traveler who lacks a certificate risks quarantine or vaccination at the border. Whenever a medical or religious reason exists for not giving a vaccine required for international travel, the physician should provide the patient with an explanatory letter typed on the physician's letterhead. The letter should be certified by the local yellow fever vaccination center.

Immunizations for Long-Term Travelers to Undeveloped Areas with Endemic or Epidemic Disease

Cholera: In areas of the world where cholera is endemic, the disease is confined largely to groups of persons living in poor socioeconomic conditions. It is very unlikely that the tourist who exercises care regarding food and drink will be at high risk for development of cholera. Cholera vaccine is only partially protective and confers short-term immunity. It should be considered only for certain high-risk travelers to highly endemic or epidemic areas. Those who receive it should be advised of its relatively poor efficacy.

Typhoid Fever: Cases of typhoid fever have been reported among travelers returning to the United States from Africa, India, and from certain countries in South America. Approximately one half of these cases have occurred among Hispanic travelers returning from Mexico, most of whom have visited small villages. Many of the *Salmonella typhi* isolates have shown plasmid-mediated resistance to commonly used antimicrobial agents.

Three types of typhoid vaccines are available for travelers. The oldest product, a killed vaccine given subcutaneously, is no longer recommended. It has been largely supplanted by an oral vaccine, a live attenuated strain of *S. typhi* administered in capsules. The newest preparation is a Vi capsular polysaccharide vaccine given by a single injection. Both new vaccines have fewer side effects and provide equivalent protection compared with the older product. Immunization is recommended for persons planning prolonged travel to developing countries known to be endemic for typhoid fever, especially those who anticipate living in areas with poor water and sanitation systems. Antimalarial chemoprophylaxis with mefloquine may blunt the immune response to the oral typhoid vaccine; mefloquine should be taken at least 24 hours before ingesting an oral vaccine capsule.

Hepatitis A: Passive immunization with immune globulin to protect against hepatitis A is recommended for travelers to areas with uncertain water and sanitation conditions. This encompasses the entire developing world, and is particularly important for persons traveling "close to the soil." The dose for adults varies; for short-term travel (3 months or less), 0.02 mL/kg to 2.0 mL given intramuscularly is sufficient. For long-term travel (more than 3 months), the dose is 0.06 mL/kg to 5.0 mL given intramuscularly. The dose should be repeated every 4 to 6 months for the duration of the period at risk. An effective hepatitis A vaccine, which will offer an alternative to immune globulin, will soon be licensed.

Hepatitis B: Hepatitis B vaccination is recommended for travelers to areas where hepatitis B is highly endemic under any of the following circumstances: 1) if travel will be for more than 6 months; (2) if sexual contact with persons from the local area is likely; and (3) if direct contact with blood or secretions of indigenous persons is anticipated, as might occur for health care workers. Travelers should be advised to avoid needle exposure, including acupuncture and tattooing, and to obtain needed dental care before traveling abroad. If time does not allow completion of a primary series of hepatitis B vaccine (6 months), an accelerated vaccination schedule has been approved for one of the hepatitis B vaccines licensed in the United States (Engerix B: with doses at 0, 30, and 60 days, and a fourth dose at 12 months if still at risk). For previously unvaccinated returning travelers who report recent high-risk events (for example, blood transfusion or unprotected high-risk sexual activity), administration of hepatitis B immune globulin within 7 days of exposure is recommended, and active immunization with hepatitis B vaccine should be started (Table 8.3).

Rabies: In many areas of the world, rabies is still endemic and can pose a substantial threat to travelers. In some developing countries, rabies vaccines derived from nervous tissue are the only preparations available, and their use is associated with an increased risk for neurologic side effects. Rather than assuming the risk of side effects from postexposure prophylaxis with such vaccines, elective pre-exposure prophylaxis with human diploid cell rabies vaccine or rabies vaccine, absorbed, should be considered for anyone planning extended travel to high-risk areas. Concurrent chloroquine prophylaxis for malaria requires that the rabies vaccine be given intramuscularly or subcutaneously because chloroquine impairs the antibody response to intradermally administered rabies vaccine.

Japanese Encephalitis: Japanese encephalitis is a mosquito-borne disease that occurs in epidemics in late summer and early autumn in temperate regions and northern tropical zones in South Asia and the Far East. In some tropical areas, the disease is endemic. The mosquito vectors are found primarily in rural areas and are present in greatest number from June through September. Prevention includes protection from mosquito bites and immunization.

Vaccination is recommended for persons planning prolonged travel (more than 1 month) to endemic areas during the transmission season, especially those visiting rural areas or sleeping in unscreened quarters. Japanese encephalitis vaccine is a killed virus vaccine. For adults, a primary series consists of three doses (1.0 mL each) given subcutaneously on days 0, 7, and 30. Possible allergic (like serum sickness) reactions with generalized urticaria and angioedema have occurred after immunization. These reactions occurred over a time range from minutes to as long as 10 days after the inoculation. Therefore, patients should have ready access to medical care during the 10 days after receiving Japanese B encephalitis vaccine.

Tuberculosis: For anyone who anticipates prolonged residence in an area highly endemic for tuberculosis, a tuberculin skin test is indicated before departure and after return. This is especially important for persons with negative results of tuberculin skin tests and a high degree of exposure (for example, health care workers and Peace Corps personnel). Bacille Calmette-Guérin vaccine is seldom indicated for adults, including foreign travelers. However, it may be indicated for tuberculin-negative infants or children who are at high risk for exposure and who lack access to medical care.

Meningococcal Infections: Meningococcal vaccine is indicated for travelers to countries with epidemic meningococcal disease. Saudi Arabia requires meningococcal vaccination for travelers entering during the annual pilgrimage to Mecca. In sub-Saharan Africa, epidemics of meningococcal disease occur frequently during the dry season (December to June). Although travelers to such areas rarely acquire meningococcal infection, the vaccine should be considered if prolonged contact with the residents is anticipated. The meningococcal vaccine available in the United States is quadrivalent, A, C, Y, W-135 vaccine. Serogroup A is the most common cause of epidemics outside the United States, but serogroup C, and, less frequently, serogroup B can also cause epidemic disease.

Plague: The traveler's risk for acquiring plague is so low that immunization is not recommended, except in rare instances in which prolonged residence in highly endemic areas is expected.

Health Maintenance

Pretravel Preparations

The goals of the pretravel office visit are 1) to anticipate medical problems that might arise during travel; 2) to obtain baseline information (for example, weight and tuberculin skin test results) that might be useful later; 3) to give indicated immunizations; 4) to answer questions and to educate patients regarding precautions related to food, drink, and sexual activity; 5) to instruct patients in self-administration of certain medications (for example, malaria prophylaxis and anti-diarrheal agents); and 6) to provide assurance to the physician that the underlying illnesses will be managed appropriately during the sojourn.

Special attention should be given to minor medical problems, especially eye, ear, nose, throat, and dental complaints, that, if left unattended, could become more serious and cause travel to be postponed or canceled. The patient should have an adequate supply of any necessary prescription medications (especially narcotic analgesics and other controlled substances), needles, and syringes and should be given a letter explaining their necessity. Patients who wear eyeglasses should carry an extra pair and a copy of the lens prescription. A "Medic-Alert" bracelet is recommended for patients with diabetes, epilepsy, or other potentially emergent medical conditions. The traveler's medical kit should be reviewed to determine the need for first-aid items, sunscreens, insect repellents, analgesics, antipyretics, antiemetics, and other medications relevant to underlying health needs.

Precautionary Measures

Food: Food is a primary source of enteric pathogens of all types. Enterotoxigenic *Escherichia coli* is a prominent cause of travelers' diarrhea. Other important agents include parasites (for example, *Giardia lamblia*), viruses (such as hepatitis A), and other bacteria (*Campylobacter, Shigella,* and *Salmonella,* for example). Because all of these pathogens are heat sensitive, travelers should be advised to eat hot cooked food. They should avoid salads, fruits that cannot be peeled after washing, foods that require considerable handling after cooking, and desserts that have been kept at room temperature for prolonged periods.

Drink: Beverages are another source of enteric pathogens. Those considered safe include hot drinks (for example, soups, coffee, and tea), carbonated beverages, beer, and wine. Iced beverages should be avoided in areas where water might be contaminated. Use of a straw or drinking directly from the can or bottle is advised if the glassware appears unclean. Boiled water or bottled carbonated water is preferred for brushing teeth. For travelers to remote areas, details of halogen treatment of contaminated water can be found in the previously cited booklet *Health Information for International Travel.*

Insect Protection: Mosquitos and flies are vectors for many parasites, including *Plasmodia, Filaria, Trypanosomes,* and *Leishmania,* and for certain bacteria and viruses. Travelers to tropical areas where insect-borne diseases are endemic should take long-sleeved clothing and an adequate supply of insect repellent containing 30% diethylmetatoluamide. Special care should be taken between dusk and dawn, the main hours for transmission of malaria. Many hotels will have adequate screens and mosquito netting, but the tourist who is traveling to more secluded areas may wish to bring mosquito netting. A spray can of insecticide is often useful.

Sexual Activity: Recognizing that unprotected sexual activity can transmit the human immunodeficiency virus and hepatitis B virus infections in developing countries has heightened the concern of travelers regarding sexually transmitted diseases. If abstinence is unlikely, hepatitis B immunization and "safer" sexual practices, especially the use of condoms, should be emphasized.

Malaria Chemoprophylaxis

Malaria is caused by infection with one or more of the four species of human *Plasmodium: falciparum, vivax, ovale,* and *malariae.* Transmitted by the bite of an infected female anopheline mosquito, malaria is undergoing a resurgence in many parts of the world. The disease occurs primarily in tropical and subtropical regions of Africa, Asia, Central and South America, and Oceania. Approximately 1100 cases of malaria among travelers are reported in the United States each year.

Specific recommendations for malaria chemoprophylaxis are influenced by several factors, including the susceptibility of *P. falciparum* to chloroquine and Fansidar in different geographic areas; seasonal variation in the risk for exposure; and local malaria-free regions (usually urban or mountainous areas) within a country. Drugs used to prevent *P. falciparum* malaria in areas of known chloroquine resistance are listed in Table 7.1. Chemoprophylaxis with all agents except doxycycline should begin 1 to 2 weeks before entering these areas to ensure adequate blood levels and to evaluate potential side effects. Chemoprophylaxis should continue during the period of malaria exposure and for 4 weeks thereafter. Current information on the occurrence of malaria in specific countries and on antimalarial chemoprophylaxis can

TABLE 7.1.   Drugs Used for Prophylaxis of Chloroquine-resistant Malaria

Drug	Prophylactic Dose*	
	Adult	**Pediatric**
Chloroquine phosphate (Aralen)	500 mg salt once a week	8.3 mg/kg salt once a week
Mefloquine (Lariam)	250 mg per week	15–19 kg: 1/4 tab per week 20–30 kg: 1/2 tab per week 31–45 kg: 3/4 tab per week >45 kg: 1 tab per week
Doxycycline	100 mg/d	>8 y, 2 mg/kg per day
Proguanil (Paludrine)	200 mg/d in combination with weekly chloroquine	<2 y, 50 mg/d 2–6 y, 100 mg/d 7–10 y, 150 mg/d > 10 y, 200 mg/d
Primaquine	15 mg/d base once per day for 14 days or 45 mg base once a week for 8 weeks	0.3 mg/kg base once per day for 14 days or 0.9 mg/kg base once a week for 8 weeks

* All medications are taken orally. The pediatric dose should not exceed the adult dose.
  All medications are taken as a single dose.

be obtained from the Centers for Disease Control and Prevention by calling 404-332-4555.

Chemoprophylaxis for Travel to Areas without Significant Risk for Exposure to Chloroquine-resistant *P. falciparum:* For the average traveler to areas without significant risk for exposure to chloroquine-resistant *P. falciparum*, chloroquine phosphate (500 mg salt once weekly) is the primary chemoprophylactic agent. It is considered safe in the dose used to prevent malaria and is considered safe for use by pregnant women. Chloroquine can interfere with the antibody response to intradermally (but not intramuscularly) administered human diploid cell rabies vaccine.

Because areas with chloroquine-sensitive *P. falciparum* are diminishing, more complex regimens for malaria chemoprophylaxis are usually required.

Chemoprophylaxis for Travel to Areas with Known Chloroquine-Resistant *P. falciparum:*

Mefloquine (Lariam): This antimalarial agent is the preferred prophylactic drug for travelers to areas where chloroquine-resistant malaria occurs. It has a structure similar to quinine and is effective against both chloroquine- and Fansidar-resistant *P. falciparum*. Adverse reactions to mefloquine are infrequent at prophylactic doses (250 mg given once a week). Mefloquine is not recommended for use by travelers with a known hypersensitivity to the drug, pregnant women, children weighing less than 15 kg, or travelers with a history of seizure disorder or psychosis. Mefloquine is not recommended for persons with cardiac conduction abnormalities, but may be used in persons concurrently on beta-blockers for other reasons.

Doxycycline: For those travelers unable to take mefloquine, doxycycline (100 mg given once a day) is an alternative regimen for travel to areas where chloroquine-resistant *P. falciparum* can be acquired. It is the drug of choice for travelers to forested regions along the Thai-Cambodia and Thai-Burmese borders because of reports of mefloquine-resistant *P. falciparum.*

Because of its short half-life, doxycycline prophylaxis can begin 1 or 2 days before entering an infected area. The traveler should be cautioned about possible side effects of tetracycline, including photosensitivity reactions, yeast vaginitis, and antibiotic-associated diarrhea. Doxycycline is contraindicated in pregnancy and for children younger than 8 years.

Chloroquine and Proguanil (Paludrine): Proguanil is a dihydrofolate reductase inhibitor not commercially available in the United States. However, it is available in Europe and in some areas where chloroquine-resistant *P. falciparum* is found. Chloroquine (500 mg given once a week) and Proguanil (200 mg given daily) together should only be prescribed when use of the more effective agents, mefloquine or doxycycline, is contraindicated. Proguanil is considered a safe drug that causes only minor gastrointestinal reactions. Chemoprophylaxis with chloroquine and proguanil is considered safe for pregnant women.

Presumptive Therapy: Presumptive treatment for malaria with a single dose (three tablets) of pyrimethamine-sulfadoxine (Fansidar) should only be considered if a febrile illness occurs and medical care is not available within 24 hours. This should only be a temporary measure until proper medical care can be obtained. Although Fansidar has been associated with severe mucocutaneous reactions when used as weekly chemoprophylaxis, a single treatment dose is considered safe. However, it should not be taken by travelers allergic to sulfonamides.

Primaquine Prophylaxis To Prevent Relapses of *P. vivax* and *P. ovale* Infections: Unlike *P. falciparum* and *P. malariae,* infections caused by *P. vivax* and *P. ovale* can persist in the liver and cause relapses as long as 4 years after cessation of chemoprophylaxis. Because primaquine can induce hemolysis in persons with glucose-6-phosphate-dehydrogenase deficiency, and because

malaria caused by *P. vivax* and *P. ovale* is usually not severe, primaquine prophylaxis is generally reserved for persons who have had prolonged exposure
to areas where malaria is endemic. Relapses can be prevented by treatment
of the liver stage of infection with primaquine (15 mg base daily) for 14
days after leaving an area endemic for *P. vivax* and *P. ovale*. Primaquine should
not be used in pregnant women.

Travelers' Diarrhea

Diarrhea develops in approximately one third of travelers to developing
countries. Precautions regarding food and drink can reduce but not eliminate the risk for disease. Because diarrhea is usually mild and because of
public health concerns about widespread antibiotic use, daily antimicrobial prophylaxis is not routinely recommended. However, antimicrobial
chemoprophylaxis with trimethoprim-sulfamethoxazole or one of the
quinolones is effective and may be recommended for travelers, especially
those in whom the consequences of diarrheal illness would be particularly
severe and persons who are business travelers or on tight travel schedules.
Although somewhat less effective, bismuth subsalicylate (Pepto-Bismol) tablets
can be used to prevent diarrheal illness for periods of risk less than 3 weeks.

Fluid and electrolyte balance can be maintained by drinking fruit juices
and caffeine-free soft drinks and eating salted crackers. Alcohol and caffeine-
containing beverages should be avoided. For patients with moderate to severe
diarrhea, oral rehydration solutions, such as those developed by the World
Health Organization, are recommended. Commercially produced packets
of standard oral rehydration solution are available throughout the developing world. The contents of each packet should be added to the appropriate volume of boiled or treated water. Unconsumed solution should be
discarded after 12 hours if it is held at room temperature.

Diphenoxylate or loperamide given to patients with no blood in the stool
and without high fever can bring rapid relief of abdominal cramps and diarrhea. For persons with evidence of inflammatory diarrhea, antiperistaltic
drugs are not advised. Bismuth subsalicylate (Pepto-Bismol) can be effective, but it acts more slowly.

After two or more loose stools accompanied by symptoms, consideration should be given to a short course (usually 3 days) of antimicrobial therapy with trimethoprim-sulfamethoxazole, trimethoprim alone, or one of
the quinolones. The quinolones offer the broadest spectrum of activity against
the bacterial causes of travelers' diarrhea. Medical attention should be sought
if diarrhea persists and is accompanied by substantial fluid loss, fever, or blood
or mucus in the stool.

8.

Clinical Issues Regarding Specific Vaccines

Cholera

Cholera is an acute diarrheal illness caused by *Vibrio cholerae* O group 1. The cholera toxin causes excessive enteric losses of fluids and electrolytes but does not cause inflammation. Even severe cases usually respond quickly to volume and electrolyte replacement given orally or parenterally. Antibiotic therapy is of secondary importance. The disease is acquired primarily by ingestion of heavily contaminated water or food. In addition to the long-term problems of endemic and epidemic cholera in Asia and Africa, South and Central America have had severe cholera epidemics in recent years. Cholera occurs most commonly when conditions of crowding and poverty exist. Cholera occurring in tourists has been rare.

Vaccine and Clinical Effectiveness

Cholera vaccine is a sterile suspension of phenol-killed *V. cholerae*. Each milliliter contains eight units of each of the two serotype antigens (OGAWA and INABA), which is roughly equivalent to 4×10^9 organisms. It should be stored at temperatures between 2 and 8 °C.

Although antibodies develop in most persons who receive cholera vaccine, the vaccine is only partially protective against clinical disease for 3 to 6 months after immunization. The vaccine does not prevent disease transmission.

Indications

Cholera vaccine is not routinely recommended for travelers because cholera occurs only rarely among travelers, the vaccine is only marginally effective, and the disease is relatively easy to treat. For these reasons, the World Health Organization no longer recommends cholera vaccination for travel to or from cholera-endemic areas. No country lists a cholera vaccination requirement, although travelers report encounters with local authorities who still request documentation of cholera vaccination. For such persons, a single 0.2-mL intradermal dose is sufficient to satisfy local requirements. Whether clear-cut indications for a complete primary series exist is debatable. A primary series is offered only to individuals who work and live in highly endemic areas that have less-than-adequate sanitary conditions and to those persons with compromised gastric defense mechanisms (for example, antacid therapy, previous surgery for gastric or duodenal ulcer, or achlorhydria).

Administration

In adults, a primary series of cholera vaccination consists of two doses (0.5 mL) given subcutaneously or intramuscularly at least 1 week apart, preferably 1 or more months apart. Alternatively, two doses can be given intradermally. The dosage for intradermal vaccination is smaller (0.2 mL), and reaction rates are predictably lower. Booster doses can be given every 6 months. Some studies indicate that lower-than-normal antibody responses to both vaccines develop in persons given yellow fever and cholera vaccines either simultaneously or within 3 weeks of each other. Unless there are time constraints, cholera and yellow fever vaccines should be administered at a minimal interval of 3 weeks; if this is not possible, they should be given simultaneously.

Adverse Reactions, Precautions, and Contraindications

Vaccination often results in 1 or 2 days of pain, erythema, and induration at the site of injection. These local reactions can be accompanied by fever, malaise, and headache. Serious reactions to cholera vaccine are rare.

No information exists on the safety of cholera vaccine given to women during pregnancy. However, it is prudent, on theoretical grounds, to avoid vaccinating pregnant women.

Revaccination

If a person has a serious reaction to cholera vaccination, reimmunization is not advised. The intradermal dose (0.2 mL) is an effective booster for persons 5 years and older.

Unresolved Issues

The available cholera vaccine probably will never be widely used in developed countries. However, the search for an effective, long-lasting vaccine continues to be important for countries where cholera is still a significant cause of death. Several orally administered vaccines are being evaluated, including subunit vaccines.

Haemophilus influenzae Type b

In the United States, *Haemophilus influenzae* type b is an uncommon cause of invasive disease in adults. Although *H. influenzae* organisms colonize in the respiratory tract and can cause otitis media and bronchitis, they are almost always nontypeable (nonencapsulated), and the infections they cause are not preventable by *H. influenzae* type b vaccination. Historically, 85% of invasive disease has occurred in children younger than 5 years, but with effective pediatric immunization programs against *H. influenzae* type b, the incidence of disease in young children has plummeted. Invasive disease can occur as meningitis, epiglotitis, cellulitis, septic arthritis, osteomyelitis, pericarditis, pneumonia, and sepsis. Persons with the human immunodeficiency virus (HIV) are at somewhat higher risk for acquiring invasive disease.

Vaccine and Clinical Effectiveness

A few studies found immunogenicity of *H. influenzae* type b vaccine in adults, but no studies have examined vaccine efficacy in the small groups of adults who might be at risk for invasive disease. The first vaccine was licensed in the United States in 1985. This vaccine was composed of the *H. influenzae* type b capsular polysaccharide polyribosyl-ribitol-phosphate (PRP). Four conjugate vaccines were licensed since then. These conjugate vaccines are more antigenic and more protective than PRP vaccine in children younger than 2 years.

Indications

No data document the effectiveness of PRP or *H. influenzae* type b conjugate vaccines in older children (5 years or older) and adults, including those with underlying conditions (for example, splenectomy, sickle cell disease, Hodgkin disease and other hematologic neoplasms, and immunosuppression) associated with increased susceptibility to infection with encapsulated bacteria. Nonetheless, a theoretical argument can be made for giving *H. influenzae* type b conjugate vaccine to such patients, including adults. Because the vaccine is safe and well tolerated, physicians may wish to consider using it on an individual basis. However, the conjugate vaccine should not be given to prevent recurrent sinusitis and bronchitis in adults. *Haemophilus influenzae* organisms associated with these conditions are almost always nontypeable, nonencapsulated strains that are not affected by antibody to *H. influenzae* type b.

Vaccination against *H. influenzae* type b is not necessary for health care personnel and day-care workers who frequently encounter children with invasive disease. In households with another unvaccinated child younger than 4 years and in day-care center classrooms with another unvaccinated child younger than 2 years, rifampin should be given to all contacts, including adults. The rifampin dosage is 20 mg/kg once daily (maximum daily dose,

600 mg) for 4 days. Pregnant women should not be given rifampin prophylaxis.

Administration, Adverse Reactions, Precautions and Contraindications, and Revaccination

When used in older children and adults, *H. influenzae* type b conjugate vaccine should be administered as a single dose (0.5 mL) intramuscularly. In children, mild local side effects occur infrequently, appear within 24 hours, and subside rapidly. More severe systemic febrile reactions are uncommon, and no long-term adverse consequences have been reported. Reaction rates with *H. influenzae* type b conjugate vaccines are similar to those with PRP vaccine. Revaccination of children and adults with the conjugate vaccines is not recommended.

Unresolved Issues

New *H. influenzae* type b conjugate vaccines are being developed. Use of these and current vaccines in adults will require a better understanding of the occurrence of invasive disease in groups of patients with conditions that might predispose them to infection and vaccine efficacy studies in these groups.

Hepatitis B

Hepatitis B virus (HBV) is a major cause of acute and chronic hepatitis in the United States. The average lifetime risk of HBV infection is 5%, but it may approach 100% for persons with many risk factors. It is estimated that 200 000 to 300 000 cases occur each year in the United States. Most HBV infections occur in young adults. Of these, jaundice develops in 25%; approximately 15 000 are hospitalized, and several hundred die of fulminant hepatitis. Approximately 5% to 10% of infected adults become long-term HBV carriers (seropositive for hepatitis B surface antigen [HBsAg] for 6 months or longer). Approximately 1 to 1.25 million such carriers live in the United States. Chronic active hepatitis develops in as many as 25% of carriers, often leading to death from cirrhosis or hepatocellular carcinoma.

The risk of HBV infection is determined by many lifestyle, occupational, and environmental factors. Those at increased risk include persons with multiple heterosexual partners, homosexual and bisexual men, health care and public safety workers, household and sexual contacts of HBsAg carriers, and users of illicit injectable drugs, among others. Infants born to mothers who are HBsAg carriers also are at risk for acquiring HBV infection during the perinatal period. Many infants born of mothers who are hepatitis B e-antigen positive develop perinatal HBV infection, and 85% to 95% of them become long-term carriers. In the United States, researchers estimate that of the 22 000 infants born to all long-term HBsAg-carrier mothers each year, approximately 6000 become chronically infected with HBV if they do not receive hepatitis B immune globulin (HBIG) and hepatitis B vaccine soon after birth.

Vaccines

The first hepatitis B vaccine became available for use in the United States in 1982. It was prepared from human plasma derived from long-term HBsAg carriers, from which HBsAg was purified and further inactivated. Use of this plasma-derived vaccine was limited because of theoretical concern that it could transmit HIV infection. However, extensive laboratory, clinical, and epidemiologic studies convincingly showed no risk for acquiring HIV infection from plasma-derived hepatitis B vaccine.

In 1986, a genetically engineered hepatitis B vaccine became available. This recombinant DNA vaccine (from Merck Sharp & Dohme, West Point, Pennsylvania) is prepared in yeast cells into which a plasmid containing the gene for HBsAg has been inserted. A second recombinant vaccine (from SmithKline Beecham) was licensed in 1989. Both recombinant vaccines are subunit HBsAg vaccines that are free of even the theoretical concern of contamination with HIV or other viruses. They replaced the plasma-derived vaccine (which is no longer produced in the United States) for all indications.

Hepatitis B Immune Globulin

Hepatitis B immune globulin is prepared from plasma obtained from donors who have a high titer of antibody to hepatitis B surface antigen (anti-HBs) but no HBsAg or antibody to HIV. Hepatitis B immune globulin preparations have an anti-HBs titer of 1:100 000 or more as measured by radioimmunoassay. In contrast, standard immune globulin preparations have an anti-HBs titer of 1:100 to 1:1000, and their protective efficacy is uncertain.

Clinical Effectiveness

A series of three doses of plasma-derived hepatitis B vaccine leads to protective levels ($\geq$10 mIU/mL) of antibody (anti-HBs) in more than 90% of healthy young adults (Table 8.1). In randomized, controlled trials among homosexually active men, hepatitis B vaccine has been shown to be 80% to 95% effective in preventing HBV infection and 100% effective in those in whom an antibody response develops after vaccination. Lower seroconversion rates have been found with increasing age and when recipients smoke or are overweight. Similarly, recent studies indicate that protective levels of

TABLE 8.1. Factors Affecting Response to Hepatitis B Vaccine*

Factor	Response ($\geq$ 10 mIU/mL)
Age, *y*	
20–29	95%
30–39	90%
40–49	86%
50–59	71%
$\geq$60	47%
Renal failure	60–70%
HIV infection	50–70%
Diabetes	70–80%
Chronic liver disease	60–70%
Sex	Female > male
Obesity	Decreased in overweight persons
Smoking	Decreased in smokers (50% lower antibody titers)
Anatomic site	Decreased if vaccinated in gluteus

* HIV = human immunodeficiency virus.
  Source: Modified from Hadler SC, Margolis HS. Hepatitis B immunization: vaccine types, efficacy, and indications for immunization. In: Remington JS, Swartz MN; eds. Current Topics in Infectious Diseases 12. New York: McGraw Hill; 1991: 282-308.

antibody develop in only 50% to 70% of HIV-infected persons after hepatitis B vaccination. Vaccine response also is diminished in patients with renal failure, chronic liver disease, or diabetes mellitus. Women have slightly better response rates than do men (Table 8.1). Combined, hepatitis B vaccine and HBIG are effective in preventing perinatal HBV infection in infants born to HBV-carrier mothers.

The immunogenicity of recombinant hepatitis B vaccines is similar to that of plasma-derived vaccine, which is no longer produced in the United States. The Merck Sharp & Dohme recombinant vaccine contains 10 µg per dose; the SmithKline Beecham vaccine contains 20 µg per dose. A three-dose series of either recombinant hepatitis B vaccine is followed by protective levels of antibody in more than 95% of healthy young adults. No clinical trials have addressed the efficacy of recombinant hepatitis B vaccines in adults.

Indications

Hepatitis B vaccine is recommended for pre-exposure and postexposure prophylaxis for several groups of persons, as outlined in Tables 8.2 and 8.3.

Pre-exposure: Researchers agree that hepatitis B vaccine has been substantially underused in all populations for which it was indicated when it

TABLE 8.2.   Pre-exposure Hepatitis B Immunization

All infants

Preadolescents (starting at 10 years), Adolescents, Young Adults

Striving to protect as many persons as possible, immunizing these young people will protect them before they become sexually active or adopt other lifestyles exposing them to risk

Persons with Occupational Risk

Now defined by the Occupational Safety and Health Administration, this includes health care workers and many public service workers. For persons in health care fields, vaccination should be completed during training before students encounter blood

Persons with Lifestyle Risk

Heterosexual persons with multiple partners (more than 1 partner in the preceding 6 months) or any sexually transmitted disease, homosexual and bisexual men, injecting drug users

Special Patient Groups

Hemophiliac persons
Hemodialysis patients

Environmental Risk Factors

Household and sexual contacts of hepatitis B virus (HBV) carriers, clients and staff of institutions for the developmentally disabled, prison inmates, immigrants and refugees from areas where HBV is highly endemic, international travelers to HBV endemic areas who are health care workers, who will reside there more than 6 months or anticipate sexual contact with local persons

---

became available more than 10 years ago. In response to this, it is recommended that all infants receive hepatitis B vaccine routinely as part of their childhood immunization series. The eventual goal of this effort is to interrupt the transmission of HBV. However, because most HBV infections occur in young adults, it is clear that major benefits will not be realized for many years. Thus, immunization of preadolescents (starting at age 10 years), all adolescents, college students, and young adults is now emphasized. In addition, the vaccine should be actively recommended to persons with multiple sex partners, homosexual and bisexual men, and others with environmental risk factors or medical conditions such as hemophilia (Table 8.2). The Occupational Safety and Health Administration now mandates that employers offer vaccine at no cost to all health care workers, public safety personnel, and others who may be occupationally exposed to blood.

The decision to vaccinate persons at risk for acquiring HBV infection frequently includes consideration of whether to screen for susceptibility before vaccination. The decision to screen is based on the costs of vaccination and testing, which are relatively constant, and the expected prevalence of pre-existing immunity, which varies depending on the group tested. Although no definitive guidelines can be given, screening groups at highest risk for HBV infection (for example, homosexual men) generally is cost-effective,

TABLE 8.3. Postexposure Prophylaxis for Hepatitis B*

Exposure	Hepatitis B Immune Globulin	Hepatitis B Vaccine
Perinatal	0.5 mL IM within 12 hours of birth	0.5 mL† IM within 12 hours of birth (no later than 7 days), and at 1 and 6 months‡; test for HBsAg and anti-HBs at 12 to 15 months
Sexual	0.06 mL kg IM within 14 days of sexual contact; a second dose should be given if the index patient remains HBAg-positive after 3 months and hepatitis B vaccine was not given initially	1.0 mL IM at 0, 1, and 6 months for homosexual and bisexual men and regular sexual contacts of persons with acute and chronic hepatits B
Percutaneous: exposed person unvaccinated		
Source known HBsAg-positive	0.06 mL/kg IM within 24 hours	1.0 mL IM within 7 days, and at 1 and 6 months§
Source known, HBsAg status not known	Test source for HBsAg; if source is positive, give exposed person 0.06 mL/kg IM once within 7 days	1.0 mL IM within 7 days, and at 1 and 6 months§
Source not tested or unknown	Nothing required	1.0 mL IM within 7 days, and at 1 and 6 months
Percutaneous: exposed person vaccinated		
Source known HBsAg-positive	Test exposed person for anti-HBs‖. If titer is protective, nothing is required; if titer is not protective, give 0.06 mL/kg within 24 hours	Review vaccination status¶
Source known, HBsAg status now known	Test source for HBsAg and exposed person for anti-HBs. If source is HBsAg-negative, or if source is HBsAg-positive but anti-HBs titer is protective, nothing is required. If source is HBsAg-positive and anti-HBs titer is not protective or if exposed person is a known nonresponder, give 0.06 mL/kg IM within 24 hours. A second dose of hepatitis B immune globulin can be given 1 month later if a booster dose of hepatitis B vaccine is not given.	Review vaccination status¶
Source not tested or unknown	Test exposed person for anti-HBs. If anti-HBs titer is protective, nothing is required. If anti-HBs titer is not protective, 0.06 mL/kg may be given along with a booster dose of hepatitis B vaccine	Review vaccination status¶

* HBsAg = hepatitis B surface antigen; anti-HBs = antibody to hepatitis B surface antigen; IM = intramuscularly; SRU = standard ratio units.
† Each 0.5-mL dose of recombinant hepatitis B vaccine contains 5 μg (Merck, Sharp & Dohme) or 10 μg (SmithKline Beecham) of HBsAg.
‡ If hepatitis B immune globulin and hepatitis B vaccine are given simultaneously, they should be given at separate sites.
§ If hepatitis B vaccine is not given, a second dose of hepatitis B immune globulin should be given 1 month later.
‖ Anti-HBs titers less than 10 SRU by radioimmunoassay or negative by enzyme immunoassay indicate lack of protection. Testing the exposed person for anti-HBs is not necessary if a protective level of antibody has been shown within the previous 24 months.
¶ If the exposed person has not completed a three-dose series of hepatitis B vaccine, the series should be completed. Test the exposed person for anti-HBs. If the antibody level is protective, nothing is required. If an adequate antibody response in the past is shown on retesting to have declined to an inadequate level, a booster dose (1.0 mL) of hepatitis B vaccine should be given. If the exposed person has inadequate an adequate antibody response in the past is shown on retesting to have declined to an inadequate level, a booster dose (1.0 mL) of hepatitis B vaccine should be given. If the exposed person has inadequate

unless the costs of testing are very high. For groups with moderate risk, including most health care workers, the cost-effectiveness of screening is marginal. For groups with a low prevalence of HBV serologic markers, including health care workers in training, screening is not cost-effective.

Postexposure Management: Postexposure prophylaxis for persons with percutaneous or mucous membrane exposure to blood or secretions known to be HBsAg positive or who have been bitten by an HBV carrier is outlined in Table 8.3. When HBIG is indicated, it should be administered as soon as possible. The value of HBIG given more than 7 days after exposure is unclear. All susceptible persons, whose sex partners have acute HBV infection or whose sex partners are HBsAg carriers, should receive a single dose of HBIG (0.06 mL/kg) and should begin the hepatitis B vaccine series.

Prenatal Screening: Prenatal screening of pregnant women for HBsAg will identify those whose infants should receive perinatal prophylaxis with hepatitis B vaccine and HBIG. Previous recommendations limited testing to certain high-risk groups, but these guidelines identified only 35% to 65% of HBV-carrier mothers. Serious problems also were encountered in the implementation of these guidelines, including lack of knowledge among health care workers of the risks for perinatal HBV transmission and the recommended screening and treatment procedures, and poor communication among persons providing care to HBV-infected mothers, their infants, and the mothers' sex partners.

Routine testing of all pregnant women is now recognized as the only strategy that will effectively control perinatal HBV infection in the United States. Current recommendations call for inclusion of HBsAg testing as part of routine prenatal care. Repeated testing later in pregnancy is unnecessary unless acute HBV infection or continued high-risk behavior (for example, parenteral drug use) is suspected. Testing for other markers of HBV infection is not necessary. Careful coordination of the activities of those providing prenatal care, hospital-based obstetrical service, and pediatric well-baby care is essential to ensure that when HBV-positive mothers are identified, their infants receive adequate prophylactic treatment and follow-up care.

Administration

Hepatitis B vaccination requires a three-dose series (1.0 mL each given intramuscularly), with the second dose given at 1 month and the third dose at 6 months. The individual dose for normal adults is 10 µg of the Merck Sharp & Dohme vaccine (Recombivax HB) and 20 µg of the SmithKline Beecham vaccine (Engerix-B) (Table 8.4). The SmithKline Beecham

TABLE 8.4.   Recommended Doses of Currently Licensed Hepatitis B Vaccines*

Group	Recombivax HB Dose[†]		Engerix-B Dose[†]	
	μg	mL	μg	mL
Infants of HBsAg-negative mothers and children <11 years old	2.5	0.5	10	0.5
Infants of HBsAg-positive mothers; prevention of perinatal infection	5	0.5	10	0.5
Children and adolescents 11 to 19 years old	5	0.5	20	1.0
Adults ≥20 years old	10	1.0	20	1.0
Dialysis patients and other immunocompromised persons	40	1.0[‡]	40	2.0[§]

* HB = hepatitis B; HBs-Ag = hepatitis B surface antigen.
[†] Both vaccines are routinely administered in a three-dose series. Engerix-B has also been licensed for a four-dose series administered at 0, 1, 2, and 12 months.
[‡] Special formulation.
[§] Two 1-mL doses administered at one site, in a four-dose schedule at 0, 1, 2, and 6 months.

preparation is also licensed for use with an alternative four-dose schedule (at 0, 1, 2, and 12 months) for postexposure prophylaxis or for more rapid induction of immunity. However, no clear-cut evidence proves that this regimen offers greater protection than the standard schedule. Patients receiving hemodialysis and those who are immunosuppressed require larger doses of vaccine (40 μg compared with 10 μg to 20 μg each), and the manufacturers provide special vaccine packaging for such use. Adolescents require only half the usual adult dose (Table 8.4).

Hepatitis B vaccine should be given in the deltoid muscle; injection in the buttock often leads to deposition of the vaccine in fat rather than in muscle, and substantially fewer persons have an adequate antibody response after intragluteal injection. For intramuscular administration of vaccine to patients who are obese, a 1 or 1.5 inch needle may be necessary to ensure that the injection is truly intramuscular.

Several studies have compared the antigenicity of intradermal with that of intramuscular vaccination. Intradermal vaccination often results in a lower frequency of protective levels of antibody. Hepatitis B vaccine is not licensed for intradermal use. If used, it should be accompanied by postvaccination testing for anti-HBs response and revaccination of persons who do not respond using the intramuscular route.

Both recombinant hepatitis B vaccines should be stored at 2 to 6 °C (36 to 43 °F) because freezing destroys their potency.

The usual dosage of HBIG for adults is 0.06 mL/kg (maximum dose, 5.0 mL) administered intramuscularly. Infants who are given perinatal HBIG prophylaxis should receive 0.5 mL intramuscularly. Hepatitis B immune globulin should not be administered intravenously.

Adverse Reactions

Recombinant hepatitis B vaccines are derived from only the HBsAg portion of the viral genome and do not contain potentially infectious viral DNA or complete virus particles.

The vaccines can produce mild soreness at the injection site in 15% to 20% of persons, which lasts 1 to 2 days. Fewer persons experience mild constitutional symptoms. Careful epidemiologic studies showed that no severe acute or chronic adverse reactions, including neurologic conditions such as Guillain-Barré syndrome, can be clearly attributed to hepatitis B vaccination. Also, no serious adverse reactions have been associated with the small residual amount of yeast-cell protein in the recombinant vaccine.

Immune globulin preparations, including HBIG, are very safe. Transient rash or low-grade fever occurs in fewer than 3% of recipients. Neither HBIG nor immune globulin transmit HBV infection. Similarly, extensive laboratory and epidemiologic studies showed that HBIG and immune globulin do not transmit HIV infection.

Precautions and Contraindications

Recombinant hepatitis B vaccines are inactivated preparations and cannot cause HBV infection. Pregnancy is not a contraindication to vaccinating women who are at high risk for infection. Pregnancy also is not a contraindication to receiving HBIG.

Management of Nonresponding Patients

After a three-dose primary series, postvaccination serologic testing is advised only for persons whose subsequent clinical management depends on knowledge of their immune status (for example, health care workers, patients receiving dialysis, and infants born to HBsAg-positive mothers). Beginning at age 30 years, an inverse relationship between antibody response and age is found (Table 8.1). Therefore, the Task Force on Adult Immunization recommends that, in vaccine recipients who are 30 years or older or who have other conditions associated with impaired vaccine response (Table 8.1), postimmunization serologic testing for HBsAb should be performed 1 to 6 months after completing the three-dose series. Persons who have not had an immunologic response after completing a hepatitis B vaccination series should receive up to three additional doses of vaccine at 1- to 2-month intervals, with serologic assessment of immunologic response after each dose.

Approximately 20% of nonresponding persons will produce antibody after one additional vaccine dose; 30% to 50% will respond after three additional doses. After 6 doses, further attempts to immunize persons who persistently do not respond are unlikely to be successful. Such individuals are candidates for passive immunization with HBIG in postexposure settings (Table 8.3).

Revaccination

Follow-up of young adults who were vaccinated with plasma-derived hepatitis B vaccine demonstrated that, 7 years later, antibody titers fell to low levels in 30% to 50% of recipients. The persistence of antibody directly correlates with the peak level achieved after the third dose. Despite these findings, protection against clinical or viremic HBV infection persists for at least 10 years. Therefore, neither booster doses of hepatitis B vaccine nor routine periodic serologic testing to determine antibody status is recommended for persons with normal immune function. The possible need for booster doses after longer intervals has yet to be established. However, vaccine-induced protection may decrease more rapidly in persons receiving hemodialysis. Annual serologic testing is recommended for these patients, with revaccination of those whose antibody levels decrease to less than 10 mIU/mL.

Booster doses of hepatitis B vaccine produce a prompt anamnestic response in persons whose previous antibody levels are undetectable. The booster dose is the same (1.0 mL administered intramuscularly) as that used for each of the doses in the initial three-dose series. The incidence of mild local adverse reactions is also similar. Pregnancy is not a contraindication to booster vaccination.

Unresolved Issues

Further studies are needed on the duration of the clinical protection after vaccination with hepatitis B vaccines and the need for booster doses after defined intervals. Greater efforts are needed to implement hepatitis B vaccination programs for health care workers, especially during their early years of training. Even more important is the need to develop effective programs for reaching other high-risk groups (for example, users of illicit injectable drugs, homosexual and bisexual men, persons with multiple sexual partners, those with recently acquired sexually transmitted diseases, and prisoners). Attention also needs to be given to implementing recent recommendations for routine screening of pregnant women and appropriate treatment and prophylaxis of newborn infants of HBsAg-positive mothers as well as universal infant immunization. Finally, less expensive hepatitis B vaccines are needed to ensure wider use, not only in the United States but throughout the world.

Immune Globulins

Immune globulins are proteins produced by B lymphocytes and plasma cells. They include specific antibodies that are critical elements of the host defense system. Five major classes of immune globulin are recognized: IgG, IgA, IgM, IgD, and IgE. All immune globulin preparations are of the IgG class and contain only small amounts of the other classes, primarily IgA. The three categories of immune globulin available for clinical use are immune globulin for intramuscular use, intravenous immune globulin (IVIG), and hyperimmune globulin preparations to protect against specific diseases such as tetanus, rabies, hepatitis B, and varicella zoster.

Immune globulin for intramuscular use has long been used to treat patients with various immunoglobulin deficiency disorders and to provide effective prophylaxis against certain viral infections. Its use is restricted to intramuscular injection; if given intravenously, anaphylactic reactions can occur because of the complement-triggering activity of aggregates of immune globulin that form in vitro. There are practical limits to the amount of and frequency with which immune globulin can be injected intramuscularly. Also, effective blood levels are achieved only after 4 to 7 days, and some immune globulin may undergo proteolytic breakdown at the injection site. For these reasons, intravenous forms of immune globulin have been developed.

Six commercial IVIG preparations are licensed for use in the United States, plus one distributed by the American Red Cross (Table 8.5). All conform to World Health Organization requirements in that 1) they are derived from plasma pools collected from at least 1000 donors to ensure a broad range of antibody specificities, 2) they contain at least 90% intact IgG molecules with full Fc (fragment, crystallizable) function and normal proportions of IgG subclasses, 3) vasoactive peptides capable of eliciting vasomotor or allergic reactions are absent, and 4) they are free from risk for infection, including viral hepatitis and HIV infection.

The manufacturing processes differ among these six preparations, and the differing purification methods result in varying concentrations of IgG, IgG subfractions, and IgA. Nonetheless, the biological activity of IVIG corresponds closely to normal human IgG antibodies with respect to serum half-life; virus neutralizing, opsonizing, and intracellular killing activity (both

TABLE 8.5. Characteristics of the Preparations of Intravenous Immune Globulin Available in the United States

Brand Name	Manufacturing Process	Additives	Approximate IgA Content* (mµ/mL)	Form Supplied	Manufacturer
Gamimune N	pH 4.25, diafiltration	10% maltose	270	5 and 10% liquid, pH 4.25	Cutter Biological, Miles Laboratories
Gammagard[†]	Polyethylene glycol, DEAE-Sephadex, ultrafiltration	2% maltose, 0.2% polyethylene glycol, 0.3 mol/L glycine, 0.15 mol/L sodium chloride, 3% albumin	0.4–1.9[‡]	Lyophilized, 5%, pH 6.8	Hyland Division, Baxter Healthcare
Gammar-IV	Low-ionic-strength ethanol	5% sucrose, 2.5% albumin, 0.5% sodium chloride	20[‡]	Lyophilized, 5%, pH 7.0	Armour Pharmaceutical
IVEEGAM	Immobilized trypsin, polyethylene glycol	5% glucose, 0.3% sodium chloride, 0.5 polyethylene glycol	5[‡]	Lyophilized, 5%, pH 6.8	Immuno-US
Sandoglobulin	pH 4.0, 1:10 000 trypsin	5% or 10% sucrose (sodium chloride in diluent)	720	Lyophilized, 3% or 6%, pH 6.6	Sandoz Pharmaceutical
Venoglobulin-1	Polyethylene glycol, DEAE-Sephadex	2% D-mannitol, 1% albumin, 0.5% sodium chloride, <0.6% polyethylene glycol	24[‡]	Lyophilized, 5%, pH 6.8	Alpha Therapeutics

*Some data were obtained from: Römer J, Späth PJ, Skvaril F, Nydegger UE. Characterization of various immunoglobulin preparations for intravenous applications. II. Complement activation and binding to Staphylococcus Protein A. Vox Sang. 1982; 42:74–80; and Apfelzweig R, Piszkiewicz D, Hooper JA. Immunoglobulin A concentrations in commercial immune globulins. J Clin Immunol. 1987; 7:46–50. Values are approximate; there is a great deal of lot-to-lot variability.

[†] Another preparation, marketed by the American Red Cross, is prepared by Baxter Hyland with plasma from Red Cross volunteer donors.

[‡] Data provided by manufacturer.

Source: Modified from: Buckley RH, Schiff RI. The use of intravenous immune globulin in immunodeficiency diseases. N Engl I Med. 1991;325:111–7.

Fc and complement mediated); and antibody activity against bacterial capsular polysaccharides. Hyperimmune IVIG preparations contain, in addition, a specific antibody level that is at least five times greater than that of standard IVIG preparations.

Clinical Effectiveness and Indications

Recommendations for intramuscular use of immune globulin and for the several hyperimmune globulin preparations in the prophylaxis, and in a few instances, treatment of specific infectious diseases are outlined in Table 8.6. Immune globulin is still used to prevent measles and hepatitis A (although it is anticipated that the availability of hepatitis A vaccines will greatly reduce the use of immune globulin for this indication). In addition, HBIG, varicella zoster immune globulin, human rabies immune globulin, and tetanus immune globulin remain effective prophylactic regimens for each of these infections. Cytomegalovirus immune globulin is a hyperimmune intravenous preparation that is effective in the prophylaxis of cytomegalovirus (CMV) infection in bone marrow and solid organ transplant recipients when given alone, and is also useful with ganciclovir to treat CMV infection in such patients. When used prophylactically for a period of several months, CMV immune globulin does not diminish the frequency of CMV infections but does modify the disease and reduce the likelihood of death. Some immunologists consider high-dose intravenous immune globulin to be equivalent to CMV-IVIG in the prophylaxis and treatment of CMV infections in high-risk patients. Vaccinia immune globulin and botulinum antitoxin are available only from the Centers for Disease Control and Prevention (404-639-3670). Because smallpox vaccination programs have been discontinued, there should be no reason to use VIG to treat the dangerous complications of vaccination except in special situations such as laboratory workers and certain military personnel.

Intravenous immune globulins have supplanted intramuscular immune globulins for replacement therapy in primary immunodeficiency syndromes. It should also be noted that intravenous immune globulin may be substituted for any indication for which intramuscular immune globulin would otherwise be recommended. Recommended uses of intravenous immune globulins are outlined in Table 8.7.

Intravenous immune globulins have been found to be effective in both acute and chronic forms of idiopathic thrombocytopenic purpura. Although intravenous immune globulin preparations have not been approved for use in pregnancy, many consider these agents as the treatment of choice for severe idiopathic thrombocytopenic purpura that occurs during pregnancy.

TABLE 8.6.   Indications for Immune Globulin for the Prevention of Specific Infectious Diseases*

Infection	Indication	Preparation	Dose
Botulism	Treatment and prophylaxis of ingestor of botulinus toxin	Specific equine antibodies	Consult CDC (404-639-3670)
Cytomega-lovirus	Prophylaxis and treatment of CMV infections in organ transplant recipients	CMV-IVIG	See package insert, intravenous preparation
Diphtheria	Treatment of respiratory diphtheria	Specific equine antibody	Consult manufacturer (800-822-2463)
Hepatitis A	Family contacts; sexual contacts; institutional or day-care outbreaks	IG	0.02 mL/kg up to 2 mL
	Travelers to developing countries	IG	0.02 mL/kg up to 2 mL for short-term (less than 3 months) travel
			0.06 mL/kg up to 5 mL for long-term (3 months or longer) travel; repeat at 4 to 6 month interval
Hepatitis B	Percutaneous or mucosal exposure	HBIG	0.06 mL/kg, vaccinate with hepatitis B vaccine if at risk for repeated exposure (for example, health care workers)
	Newborns of HBsAg-positive mothers	HBIG	0.5 mL at birth, vaccinate with hepatitis B vaccine
	Sexual contacts of persons with acute or chronic hepatitis B	HBIG	0.06 mL/kg vaccinate with hepatitis B vaccine
Measles	Nonimmune contacts of acute cases exposed fewer than 6 days previously	IG	0.25 mL/kg up to 15 mL for normal hosts 0.5 mL/kg up to 15 mL for immunocompromised persons
Rabies	Persons exposed to rabid or potentially rabid animals	HRIG	20 IU/kg
Tetanus	Following significant exposure of an unimmunized person	TIG	250 units for prophylaxis
	Immediately on diagnosis of disease	TIG	3000 to 6000 units for therapy
Vaccinia	Severe reactions to vaccinia vaccination	VIG	Available only from CDC's Drug Service (404-639-3670)
Varicella zoster	Immunosuppressed or newborn contacts	VZIG	125 units per 10 kg, up to 625 units. Fractional doses are not recommended

* IG = immune globulin; HBIG = hepatitis B immune globulin; TIC = tetanus immune globulin; VZIG = varicella zoster immune globulin; HRIG = human rabies immune globulin; CMV-IVIG = cytomegalovirus intravenous immune globulin; VIG = vaccinia immune globulin. CDC = Centers for Disease Control and Prevention. Immune globulin should be administered intramuscularly, except if clearly labeled for intravenous use. *See* text for details.

TABLE 8.7. Recommended Uses of Intravenous Immune Globulins

Primary immunodeficiency syndromes
  Specific antibody deficiencies: X-linked agammaglobulinemia; common variable immunodeficiency; antibody deficiency with normal immunoglobulin levels, for example

  Combined deficiencies; severe combined immunodeficiencies (all types); Wiskott-Aldrich syndrome, ataxia-telangiectasia; short-limbed dwarfism; X-linked lymphoproliferative syndrome.

Idiopathic thrombocytopenic purpura
Chronic lymphatic leukemia
Kawasaki disease

In chronic lymphatic leukemia, intravenous immune globulins have been shown to reduce the frequency of serious infections caused by *Streptococcus pneumoniae* and *H. influenzae*. Although the measured benefit in clinical trials is statistically significant, the cost of such prophylaxis is enormous, and the overall clinical benefit in terms of quality of life is not clearly defined. A National Institutes of Health consensus conference on Kawasaki disease found sufficient evidence to establish that intravenous immune globulins were effective in preventing the development of coronary aneurysms. Intravenous immune globulin should be administered to such patients only if strict criteria for Kawasaki disease have been met.

Immune globulins have been used in a number of other ways, many of which are the subject of ongoing research (Table 8.8). Initial studies documented efficacy of IVIG in neonatal sepsis, surgical sepsis, prevention of bacterial and viral infections in HIV-infected children, in the Guillain-Barré syndrome, and related inflammatory demyelinating polyneuropathies. Other possible uses include the treatment of epilepsy and a number of autoimmune diseases, including rheumatoid arthritis, polymyositis, and systemic lupus erythematosis. Data are incomplete, and intravenous immune globulin cannot be recommended for routine clinical use in these disorders at this time.

In addition, a number of monoclonal antibody preparations, containing antibody directed against specific toxins or inflammatory mediators, are being investigated (Table 8.9). Monoclonal antibody directed at the core glycolipid of the endotoxin of gram-negative bacilli has been studied extensively, with results that are still equivocal. Other immunoglobulin preparations for treating sepsis and septic shock are being developed. All are likely to be very expensive and will raise cost-benefit issues.

TABLE 8.8.   Investigational Uses of Intravenous Immune Globulins*

Neonatal sepsis
Epilepsy
Guillain-Barré syndrome
Autoimmune diseases
   Neutropenia
   Hemolytic anemia
   Bullous pemphigoid
   Type 1 diabetes mellitus
   Myasthenia gravis
   Rheumatoid arthritis
   Polymyositis
   Systemic lupus erythematosus
Prevention of sepsis and GVH disease in bone marrow transplant
Prevention of bacterial and viral infections in HIV-infected children
Postoperative sepsis
Multiple sclerosis
Pediatric asthma

* GVH = graft-versus-host disease; HIV = human immunodeficiency virus.

Administration

The recommended dose requirements for intramuscular immune globulin preparations are well established and are shown in Table 8.6. Dose requirements for IVIG preparations are more complex. In general, serum levels after intravenous administration are related to the dose given, with doses of 100 mg/kg and 500 mg/kg resulting in increases in peak serum IgG levels of approximately 200 mg/dL and 1000 mg/dL, respectively. After 3 days, serum levels decrease by approximately 50%, and then decrease to preinfusion levels after 3 to 4 weeks. However, considerable variability is found among patients regarding serum levels achieved and their rates of decline.

In immunodeficient patients treated with IVIG, serum levels may not correlate with protection; prevention of clinical infection is still the best measure of therapeutic efficacy. Whether larger doses of IVIG (for example, 500 to 600 mg/kg given every 3 or 4 weeks) provide better protection than the commonly used dose of 300 to 400 mg/kg given approximately each month is not yet determined. Physicians should be guided by clinical observation and try to achieve trough serum IgG concentrations between 400 and 500 mg/dL.

Adverse Reactions, Precautions, and Contraindications

Physicians and the public have raised concerns that immune globulin or IVIG might transmit HIV, hepatitis virus, or both. Some lots of immune globulin produced before 1985 contained antibody to HIV, and recipients became transiently positive for HIV antibody for periods of less than 1 month. However, no evidence of viral reverse transcriptase was found in either treated patients or in immune globulin preparations. In addition, HIV-associated changes in T lymphocytes were not observed in recipients of these preparations, nor was serologic evidence of persistent HIV infection ascribed to immune globulin administration. Also, when viable HIV was added to lots of plasma undergoing Cohn ethanol fractionation, all traces of the virus were removed. Since 1985, all units of plasma used for preparing immune globulin products must be negative for the HIV antibody. These data should reassure physicians and the public that immune globulin and IVIG preparations cannot transmit HIV infection.

With the exception of two cases of hepatitis B caused by contamination of a single lot of IVIG, no other cases of hepatitis have been reported after administration of immune globulin preparations produced in the United States. In Europe, four cases of non-A, non-B hepatitis were reported after administration of IVIG, but none have been reported with licensed products in the United States.

Local reactions are common with intramuscular immune globulin, particularly when more than 2 mL are given. However, systemic reactions are uncommon, affecting only 0.1% to 0.2% of recipients. With IVIG, systemic reactions are more common, affecting 3% to 12% of recipients. Most of these reactions are not anaphylactic, but rather are probably due to the union of infused antibody and bacterial antigens in the patient. They are characterized by chills, nausea, abdominal discomfort, flushing, headache, backache, dizziness, and joint pain, and are most frequently seen in a newly

TABLE 8.9.   Investigational Monoclonal Antibodies for Treating Sepsis and Septic Shock

Antibodies Directed Against
  Endotoxin
  Bacterial exotoxins
  Tumor necrosis factor-α
  Interleukin-1
  Phospholipase A_2
  Complement fragments
  Adhesion molecules

diagnosed patient or in a patient who has chronic lung, sinus, or other types of infections. They can be avoided by decreasing the rate of infusion; by pretreating patients with salicylates, acetaminophen, or diphenhydramine; or by increasing the trough serum IgG concentration closer to the normal range. Anaphylactic reactions are rare and occur predominantly in patients with common variable immunodeficiency who have no IgA, but who do have anti-IgA antibodies, sometimes after previous exposure to blood products, including immune globulin. Therefore, treating patients with isolated IgA deficiency with immune globulin is not only ineffective but also potentially dangerous. In patients with IgA deficiency who have profound antibody deficiency, and when immune globulin therapy could be helpful, only preparations known to be very low in contaminating IgA should be used. Immune globulin preparations should be administered initially under direct medical supervision in settings where anaphylaxis can be treated immediately.

Other rare reactions to IVIG, probably idiosyncratic in nature, have included alopecia, aseptic meningitis, acute renal failure, and retinal necrosis.

Unresolved Issues

Recommendations for use of IVIG in the many disorders currently considered investigational must await further clinical studies (Table 8.8). Similarly, use of monoclonal antibody preparations directed against bacterial components or against inflammatory mediators (Table 8.9) is one of the most active areas of clinical investigation in immunobiology.

Influenza

Influenza A viruses are classified into subtypes based on their hemagglutinin (H) and neuraminidase (N) antigens. Three hemagglutinin (H1, H2, and H3) and two neuraminidase (N1 and N2) subtypes represent the major antigenic subtypes of influenza A viruses that cause widespread human disease. These antigens change progressively with time (antigenic drift), so that eventually infection or vaccination by one strain will provide little or no protection against infection by a subsequent, distantly related strain of the same subtype. Antigenic variation also occurs with influenza B viruses, although less frequently. These continuous minor antigenic changes and the occasional major antigenic change represented by the occurrence of a new subtype, account for frequent and severe outbreaks of disease.

Influenza is an acute, febrile respiratory illness, often associated with prominent constitutional symptoms, especially headache and myalgia. Full recovery may be delayed for many days or even several weeks. Because attack rates sometimes approach 20% to 30%, outbreaks of influenza disrupt community life and cause dramatic increases in the use of health care services. Elderly persons and those with certain underlying medical conditions, especially cardiopulmonary diseases, are at increased risk for experiencing more severe influenza and more complicated illness, usually secondary bacterial pneumonia. Compared with the general population, these persons are more likely to need hospital care once infected. Influenza is associated with excess mortality, with deaths increasing by 10 000 to 50 000 during epidemics. Generally, 80% to 90% of influenza-associated excess mortality occurs among persons 65 years and older. Given the increasing number of elderly persons and persons living with high-risk medical conditions, the impact of influenza will probably increase.

Vaccine

Influenza vaccine is made from egg-grown viruses that are highly purified and inactivated and cannot cause infection. Since 1976, the vaccine has contained two type A strains (H1N1 and H3N2) and one type B strain, representing the most recent influenza viruses circulating in the world and believed likely to cause disease in the United States. It is available in both whole virus and split virus (subvirion) preparations. In adults, the antigenicity and frequency of adverse reactions of the two preparations are generally similar, although in children, split virus (subvirion) vaccines have been better tolerated than whole virus preparations.

Clinical Effectiveness

The protection afforded by influenza vaccination is best correlated with the development of serum antihemagglutinin antibodies. Vaccination in younger adults is usually associated with a 70% to 90% reduction in clinical illness caused by the same or a closely related influenza virus. In older persons vaccine efficacy is often less; in nursing home residents, the vaccine may be only 30% to 40% effective in preventing clinical illness, although it is more effective in preventing pneumonia, hospitalization, and death. In residential institutions, vaccination rates of more than 80% appear to generate sufficient herd immunity that only sporadic cases of influenza, rather than outbreaks, are likely to occur. Approximately 30% to 40% of noninstitutionalized elderly persons, and approximately 10% of younger high-risk persons, receive influenza vaccine each year. More effective strategies are needed to deliver influenza vaccine to high-risk persons, health care providers, and their household contacts. Physicians and other health care providers should implement programs to ensure that persons for whom influenza vaccine is recommended are immunized. Of particular note is the fact that, in 1993, the cost of influenza immunization became reimbursable by Medicare (*see* Chapter 2, Implementation Strategies).

Indications

Influenza vaccination is indicated for all persons who are at increased risk for influenza-related complications or who, if infected, can transmit influenza to high-risk persons. Highest priority should be given to residents of nursing homes and other long-term care facilities and to adults and children (6 months or older) with chronic cardiopulmonary disorders who required regular medical care or hospitalization during the preceding year. Next in priority should be persons with chronic metabolic diseases, including diabetes mellitus, renal disease, hemoglobinopathies, or immunosuppression, who require regular medical care or who had previous hospital care, and otherwise healthy persons 65 years or older. In addition, children, adolescents, and young adults who are receiving long-term aspirin therapy should be vaccinated because they risk contracting Reye syndrome if they become infected with influenza.

Greater attention should be given to vaccinating healthy persons who, if infected with influenza virus, can transmit infection to high-risk persons. Physicians, nurses, students, and other health care workers should be immunized, especially those who have regular contact with high-risk patients in hospitals and in long-term care facilities. Providers of home care to high-risk persons and their close household contacts also should be vaccinated. Because the vaccine is considered safe for the fetus, pregnant women should be vaccinated if they have underlying high-risk medical conditions. Influenza vaccine can be given to any person who wishes to reduce the risk for influenza infection. Persons who provide essential community services may be considered for vaccination to minimize the disruption created by influenza outbreaks. Influenza vaccine should also be considered for international travelers, especially if their itinerary takes them to areas where influenza outbreaks are probable (*see* Chapter 7, Immunizations and Other Preventive Measures for International Travel).

The efficacy of influenza vaccine in highly immunocompromised patients is not known. However, because influenza may result in serious illness and complications in persons with HIV, vaccination appears to be prudent and usually results in antibody responses in many recipients. In patients with advanced HIV-related illnesses, however, vaccine response may be suboptimal or completely absent. Repeated doses of influenza vaccine have not increased the immune response in such persons.

Administration

Influenza vaccine should be administered intramuscularly, not subcutaneously or intradermally. In adults, one dose (0.5 mL) is sufficient, and both the whole or the split virus preparation are approved for use. Influenza vaccine may be given at the same time as pneumococcal, measles, mumps, rubella, *H. influenzae* type b, and oral polio vaccines.

Adverse Reactions

Influenza vaccines are inactivated preparations that do not contain infectious virus. Respiratory illnesses sometimes occur after vaccination but represent coincidental infection with unrelated agents.

The most frequent side effect of influenza vaccination is soreness at the injection site that lasts 1 or 2 days. Two types of systemic reactions have been observed. In the first type, fever, myalgia, and malaise occur 6 to 12 hours after vaccination and last 1 or 2 days. These reactions usually affect younger persons with no previous exposure to the antigens in the vaccine. The second type consists of more severe immediate hypersensitivity reactions (hives, angioedema, allergic asthma, or systemic anaphylaxis) and are rare. These reactions are probably caused by tiny amounts of residual egg protein in vaccine given to persons with a severe underlying allergy to eggs.

In 1976, swine influenza vaccination was associated with an increased frequency of Guillain-Barré syndrome in the weeks immediately after vaccination. From 1977 to 1990, no association between influenza vaccination and Guillain-Barré syndrome or other serious neurologic conditions was observed. In the 1990 to 1991 season, a small excess of reported cases of Guillain-Barré syndrome over predicted cases was observed in the 6 weeks after influenza vaccination in adults younger than 65 years. The number of cases of Guillain-Barré syndrome in adults older than 65 years was less than predicted in the same time period. The significance of these observations is not clear, but little evidence of an association with influenza vaccine exists. Although influenza vaccination can alter the hepatic clearance of several commonly used drugs (warfarin, theophylline, and phenytoin), the magnitude of these changes is not clinically significant.

Precautions and Contraindications

Influenza vaccine should not be given to those rare persons who have anaphylactic hypersensitivity to eggs. Such reactions include hives, swelling of the lips or tongue, or acute respiratory distress or collapse after eating eggs. Asthma or other allergic responses after occupational exposure to egg protein also are contraindications. Persons who eat eggs or egg-containing foods without incident can be vaccinated safely.

Minor intercurrent illness is not a contraindication to influenza vaccination. Most authorities recommend that influenza immunization be delayed in persons with an active neurologic disorder characterized by changing neurologic findings, but should be considered when the disease process has been stabilized. Influenza vaccine should not be given to patients who have had Guillain-Barré syndrome or other neurologic illnesses related to previously administered vaccine.

Revaccination

Persons for whom influenza vaccination is indicated should be revaccinated each year with the currently recommended vaccine; unused vaccine from the previous year should not be given. Physicians should establish procedures to ensure that their high-risk patients are notified each year of the need for revaccination, and such patients should be encouraged to request vaccination each fall (*see* Chapter 2, Implementation Strategies).

Antiviral Prophylaxis and Therapy

Rimantadine hydrochloride and amantadine hydrochloride are effective prophylactic and therapeutic agents against influenza A virus infection. They are not effective against influenza B virus infection. Both drugs interfere with the replication of influenza A viruses. Despite the chemical similarities of the two drugs, they differ substantially in their pharmacokinetic properties. Approximately 90% of rimantadine is metabolized by the liver before renal excretion, whereas more than 90% of amantadine is excreted unchanged by the kidneys. Amantadine has a slower rate of clearance and achieves a higher plasma concentration than does rimantadine at a similar dose. They are 70% to 90% effective when given prophylactically to healthy adults. The incidence of adverse central nervous system side effects appears to be less for rimantadine compared with amantadine at equivalent doses.

Rimantadine or amantadine prophylaxis is recommended as an adjunct to vaccination when vaccine is given after a community outbreak of influenza A occurs. The drug should be taken for 2 weeks to provide early protection until vaccine-induced antibodies appear. Rimantadine or amantadine prophylaxis is also recommended for unvaccinated household members and other caregivers who have close contact with high-risk persons in the home, and for high-risk persons for whom influenza vaccine is contraindicated. In addition, chemoprophylaxis should be considered as supplemental protection for immunodeficient persons, including those with HIV infection, who can be expected to have a suboptimal antibody response to influenza vaccination. It can also be have a suboptimal antibody response to influenza vaccination. It can also be given to anyone who wishes to avoid infection with influenza A virus.

Rimantadine or amantadine prophylaxis can be especially useful in controlling outbreaks of influenza among high-risk persons in nursing homes, other long-term care facilities, and hospitals. Once an outbreak of influenza A is recognized, consideration should be given to treating all patients, regardless of previous receipt of influenza vaccine. Influenza chemoprophylaxis should be offered to unvaccinated staff who care for high-risk patients.

Treatment of acute influenza A illness with rimantadine or amantadine can shorten the duration of fever and the severity of other symptoms in healthy adults if initiated within 24 to 48 hours of illness onset. No data are available on the efficacy of these drugs in preventing the complications of influenza A among high-risk persons. Because of possible induction of drug resistance, rimantadine or amantadine treatment of persons with influenza-like illness should be discontinued as soon as signs and symptoms resolve, generally within 3 to 5 days. To reduce the risk for emergence and spread of drug-resistant influenza A, persons receiving rimantadine or amantadine for treatment should be separated, when feasible, from persons taking these drugs for prophylaxis. Neither rimantadine nor amantadine interferes with the normal antibody response to influenza A virus infection.

Dosage recommendations for rimantadine and amantadine are given in Table 8.10.

At a dose of 200 mg per day, amantadine causes nausea, dizziness, insomnia, and difficulty with concentration in 5% to 10% of young adults. Other more serious central nervous system-related side effects, such as seizures and confusion, are less frequent, but have been encountered in elderly persons, patients with renal disease, and patients with seizure disorders. Reducing the amantadine dose to 100 mg per day appears to reduce the frequency of these side effects among such persons without compromising the prophylactic effectiveness of amantadine. Even at the 100-mg dose, as many as one third of nursing home patients may suffer adverse reactions.

In elderly persons known to have impaired renal function, or in persons who are smaller than average, the dose should be reduced further. Rimantadine dose should be reduced for patients with severe hepatic or renal dysfunction (Table 8.10). Adverse reactions to amantadine encountered in nursing home patients include psychosis, ataxia, hallucinations, seizures, congestive heart failure, and falls. Risk factors associated with severe adverse reactions have included confinement to bed or chair, multiplicity of underlying diagnoses, congestive heart failure, and elevated serum creatinine. Thus, although amantadine prophylaxis of influenza A in nursing homes may be

TABLE 8.10.   Dosage Recommendations for Amantadine and Rimantadine

Drug	Age Group, years			
	1–9	**Children ≥10**	**Adults <65**	**≥65**
Amantadine*				
Treatment	4.4 mg/kg per day up to 150 mg	100 mg bid[†]	100 mg bid	≤100 mg/d
Prophylaxis	4.4 mg/kg per day up to 150 mg	100 mg bid[†]	100 mg bid	≤100 mg/d
Rimantadine[‡]				
Treatment	NA	NA	100 mg bid	100 or 200 mg/d[§]
Prophylaxis	5 mg/kg per day up to 150 mg	100 mg bid[‖]	100 mg bid	100 or 200 mg/d[§]

* Dosage recommendations for administering amantadine to persons with creatinine clearance rates less than 30 mL/min can be found in the drug package insert.

† Children 10 years or older who weigh less than 45 kg should be given amantadine at a dose of 4.4 mg/kg per day.

‡ A reduction in dose to 100 mg/d of rimantadine is also recommended for persons with severe hepatic dysfunction or those with creatinine clearance ≤10 mL/min. Other persons with less severe hepatic or renal dysfunction taking >100 mg/d should be observed closely and the dose reduced or the drug discontinued if necessary.

§ Elderly nursing home residents should be given only 100 mg/d of rimantadine. A reduction in dose to 100 mg/d should be considered for all persons 65 years or older if they experience side effects when taking 200 mg/d. A reduction in dose to 100 mg/d is also recommended for persons with severe hepatic dysfunction and those with creatinine clearance rates ≤10 mL/min. Other persons with less severe renal insufficiency taking >100 mg/d should be observed closely and the dosage reduced if necessary.

‖ Children 10 years or older who weigh less than 45 kg should be given rimantadine at a dose of 5 mg/kg per day.

effective, its safe use requires close supervision and monitoring. Fewer adverse reactions are anticipated (but not yet proved) with rimantadine.

Unresolved Issues

Many studies show that influenza vaccination of older high-risk persons is effective in preventing illness and death. Nonetheless, influenza immunization in elderly high-risk persons is substantially less effective than in young adults, and influenza A continues to be a major cause of hospitalization and death in elderly institutionalized persons. Improved influenza vaccines for the elderly are needed, and thus the utility of live attenuated influenza virus vaccines must be determined. One possibility is to combine vaccines; there is evidence that a live attenuated vaccine, given to elderly persons with standard trivalent inactivated vaccine, provides a higher level of protection against influenza than the inactivated vaccine alone.

The relative merits of rimantadine compared with amantadine in influenza A treatment and prophylaxis must be established and the role of these drugs in influenza control needs to be better defined in clinical trials.

Information is also needed on the serologic profiles and clinical effectiveness in persons who receive influenza vaccine annually for an extended period. Evidence exists that annual immunization during a period of 5 years does not lead to any loss of protective capacity among middle-aged persons. If such studies are performed in elderly high-risk patients they should evaluate functional status, quality of life, and use of health care services. Finally, more information is needed about determinants of successful vaccination programs, including their organization, administration, incentives, and reimbursement policies, to improve the delivery of influenza vaccine to older and high-risk patients.

Japanese Encephalitis

Japanese encephalitis is a mosquito-borne arboviral infection that occurs throughout Asia, including China, Korea, Japan, and India. A small proportion of infected persons become ill. When illness occurs, however, encephalitis is severe; 25% of patients die and 50% of survivors have neurologic sequelae.

The major vertebrate hosts of the virus are the domestic pig and certain birds; thus the disease is most common in rural areas. In temperate regions, the virus is transmitted from May through September; in the tropics, mosquito populations vary with rainfall and the location of irrigation ditches, and thus transmission may occur throughout the year.

The risk for Japanese encephalitis in travelers to Asia is low. However, persons staying for an extended period and those who travel to rural areas risk greater exposure to infection. Since 1981, 10 cases of Japanese encephalitis were recognized in American travelers, 7 of which were associated with military service. The Centers for Disease Control and Prevention estimates that the risk for Japanese encephalitis in American travelers to Asia is less than 1 in 1 million. However, travelers to rural areas during transmission season may have a risk of 1 in 20 000 each week. Use of insect repellents, protective clothing, and avoidance of outdoor activities during twilight and the evening reduces the risk for infection.

Vaccine and Clinical Effectiveness

The vaccine is a formalin-inactivated product derived from infected mouse brains that was developed in Japan and has been used throughout Asia since 1954. Field trials in Thailand and China found that a two-dose schedule was 80% to 91% effective. However, immunogenicity studies in American and British persons showed that three doses were required to induce protective levels of neutralizing antibodies.

Indications

Japanese encephalitis vaccine is not recommended for all travelers to Asia, particularly those on short trips to regular tourist destinations. Individual recommendations should be based on risk. In general, the vaccine is appropriate for persons spending at least 1 month in an endemic area during the transmission season, especially if time will be spent in rural areas, and for persons taking short trips to highly endemic areas. Mosquito prevention measures are essential.

Administration, Adverse Reactions, Precautions, and Contraindications

The primary series consists of three subcutaneous doses (1.0 mL each) given on days 0, 7, and 30. A shortened schedule given on days 0, 7, and 14 can be used when necessary. Booster doses may be given after 2 years. Because of the concern about urticarial and other reactions, vaccinated persons should be observed for at least 30 minutes after inoculation. During the subsequent 10-day period, they should remain in places where medical care is available should a delayed hypersensitivity reaction occur.

Local reactions occur in about 20% of vaccinated persons and systemic symptoms of fever, headache, chills, nausea, and abdominal pain have been noted in as many as 10% of recipients. Because the vaccine is prepared in neural tissue, there have been concerns about neurologic side effects, but a causal relationship between vaccination and rare, temporally related neurologic events has not been established.

Since 1989, a new adverse reaction has been observed in which urticaria and angioedema have occurred, sometimes with respiratory distress and hypotension requiring emergent medical care. Some of these reactions occurred immediately, but surprisingly the interval between vaccination and the onset of these acute hypersensitivity reactions was often prolonged by a median of 12 hours and for as long as 9 days. Some reactions occurred only after the second or third dose of vaccine. Treatment with antihistamines and steroids has generally been successful. Persons who have a past history of urticaria may be at increased risk for these reactions. Several recent studies indicate a wide range of potential risk for hypersensitivity reactions, from 0.7 to 100 per 10 000 vaccinated persons. Surveillance of adverse reactions during a mass immunization program of 16 000 U.S. military personnel in Japan revealed the sudden death of a 21-year-old man who had received a first dose of Japanese encephalitis vaccine 60 hours earlier. The cause of death was not determined at autopsy.

The safety of vaccination for pregnant women has not been determined.

Unresolved Issues

The vaccine components producing the hypersensitivity reactions have not been identified. The appropriate interval for booster immunization has not been well studied.

Measles

Measles is a highly communicable, serious infection often complicated by otitis media or pneumonia. Encephalitis or death follows measles in approximately 1 in 1000 reported cases. The risk for encephalitis is greater in adults than in children, and after infants, the highest case-fatality rate occurs in adults. Measles during pregnancy increases the risk for spontaneous abortion, premature labor, and low birth weight.

After nearly a decade of relatively little measles activity, a resurgence of measles cases occurred in the United States from 1989 to 1991. Although the increase primarily involved young, unvaccinated children in inner-city areas, an increase in cases also occurred among adults 20 years and older, who accounted for 20% of cases and 26% of reported deaths. Among adults, colleges and other postsecondary institutions, health care settings, and international travel were important factors in exposure to measles. Coincident with intensive efforts to improve measles immunization at all levels, the incidence of measles returned to record low levels in 1993.

Vaccine and Clinical Effectiveness

Measles vaccine (licensed in 1963) is a live attenuated virus vaccine prepared in chick embryo cell culture. It produces a mild or inapparent noncommunicable infection. It is available as monovalent (measles only), as measles and rubella (MR), and measles, mumps, and rubella (MMR) vaccines. In most circumstances, MMR is preferred. A single dose of measles vaccine induces protection in approximately 95% of recipients that is probably lifelong in most people. The two-dose schedule now recommended for children and some high-risk adults is expected to provide protection for most persons who do not respond to their initial vaccinations.

Indications

Primary Immunization: Measles vaccine is indicated for all adults born after 1956 who lack documentation of immunization with live measles vaccine on or after their first birthday, physician-diagnosed measles, or laboratory evidence of immunity. In addition, persons who received live measles vaccine before their first birthdays, or within several months after administration of immune globulin (Table 1.6); those who received killed measles vaccine alone or killed measles vaccine followed within 3 months by live vaccine; or those who received a measles vaccine of unknown type between 1963 and 1967 should receive another dose of live measles vaccine. Because detailed information on childhood vaccines and illnesses is not easily available for most adults, a practical strategy is to immunize with MMR all healthy adults born after 1956.

In 1989, the Committee on Infectious Disease of the American Academy of Pediatrics and the Advisory Committee on Immunization Practices recommended a two-dose schedule for measles immunization, with the first dose given at 15 months and the second dose given during school-age years. Both doses should be given as MMR. Although the two-dose schedule is recommended for all children, it is recommended only for selected high-risk adults (*see* Revaccination below).

Postexposure Management: In general, susceptible adults who are exposed to measles should be vaccinated immediately because the vaccine is likely to be protective only if administered within 72 hours of exposure. If exposure does not result in infection, vaccination will protect against subsequent measles infection. An acceptable alternative is immune globulin, which can prevent or modify infection if given within 6 days of exposure. Immune globulin is particularly useful for patients who have contraindications to measles vaccine. Immune globulin should not be used to control measles outbreaks. The recommended dose is 0.25 mL/kg (0.5 mL/kg in immunosuppressed individuals) given intramuscularly, not to exceed 15 mL/kg, and no more than 5 mL/kg should be injected at any one site. Live measles vaccine should be given 5 months after immune globulin is administered (6 months if the 0.5-mL/kg dose is given), by which time passive measles antibodies should have disappeared.

Administration and Adverse Reactions

Measles vaccine (0.5 mL given as single antigen, MR, or MMR vaccine) should be given subcutaneously. The measles, mumps, and rubella vaccine is the preferred formulation. Whenever two doses are required, they should be separated by no less than 1 month. Adverse reactions do not appear to be age related. Fever greater than 39.4 °C (103 °F) develops in approximately 5% to 15% of recipients. This reaction generally occurs 5 to 12 days after vaccination, usually lasts 1 or 2 days, and may be associated with febrile seizures in children. Transient rashes have been reported in approximately 5% of vaccinated persons. The incidence of encephalitis after measles vaccination is lower than the observed background incidence of encephalitis of unknown cause and is much lower than that associated with naturally occurring measles.

From 40% to 55% of persons who previously received killed measles vaccine experience reactions after live measles vaccination. Most are local and sometimes are accompanied by low-grade fever lasting 1 or 2 days. Such reactions can be severe but are considerably milder than atypical measles, the illness that follows exposure to natural measles in persons who have received killed measles vaccine.

Precautions and Contraindications

Minor illness is not a contraindication to measles vaccination. In persons with severe febrile illness, measles vaccination should be postponed until after recovery. Vaccination should not be given for the 14 days before and several months after a person has received immune globulin, whole blood, or other antibody-containing blood products. (Table 1.6)

Because of the theoretical risk to the developing fetus, measles vaccine should not be given to pregnant women or to women who are considering becoming pregnant within 3 months of vaccination. Also, it should not be given to persons who are immunocompromised as a result of most immunodeficiency diseases, leukemia, lymphoma, or generalized malignancy, or to persons who are immunosuppressed as a result of therapy with corticosteroids, alkylating drugs, antimetabolites, or radiation. However, persons with leukemia who are in remission and have not received chemotherapy for at least 3 months and clinically well persons with HIV should be vaccinated against measles, if they are considered susceptible. Although measles vaccine has been safely given to HIV-infected children, there is little information regarding its safety in HIV-infected adults. The Task Force on Adult Immunization recommends that asymptomatic HIV-infected individuals should receive the measles vaccine when indicated; but for persons who have progressed to AIDS, the decision should be individualized based on the degree of immunosuppression and the likelihood of exposure to measles. Postexposure prophylaxis with immune globulin should be given strong consideration, regardless of previous history of measles or measles vaccination in immunocompromised persons.

No evidence exists that live measles vaccine exacerbates tuberculosis. Measles vaccination can temporarily suppress tuberculin reactivity; therefore, tuberculin skin testing, if indicated, should be done either on the day of vaccination or 4 to 6 weeks later.

Vaccination is not recommended for persons with a history of anaphylactic reaction after ingesting eggs or receiving neomycin. Protocols have been developed for vaccinating persons with severe egg allergy for whom the benefit of the vaccine is thought to outweigh the potential risks.

Revaccination

Revaccination, preferably with MMR, is recommended for some adults born after 1956. Protection against measles is particularly important when the risk for exposure to natural disease is increased, as occurs in postsecondary education institutions, health care settings, and during travel to areas where measles is endemic. Because one dose of measles vaccine fails to provide protection in as many as 5% of vaccinated persons, documentation of two doses of measles vaccine, physician-documented natural measles, or serologic evidence of immunity is recommended in these settings. In addition, because 29% of health care workers in whom measles developed from 1985 to 1989 were born before 1957, serious consideration should be given to assuring their immunity to both measles and rubella by immunization or serologic screening, because the consequences of transmission of these diseases in the health care setting are serious. In persons with either natural or vaccine-induced immunity, revaccination is not associated with adverse effects.

Unresolved Issues

Severe cases of measles have been reported in susceptible immunocompromised persons. Because MMR vaccine has been given without untoward incident in healthy persons infected with HIV and in persons with leukemia in remission, it is recommended for such persons. The risks and benefits of measles vaccine in other conditions associated with immunosuppression are not known.

Meningococcal Infections

Meningococcal disease is endemic throughout the world, but sometimes epidemics occur. In the United States, meningococcal infections usually occur as isolated cases or, infrequently, as small localized outbreaks. One third of cases affect persons 20 years or older. Most cases are caused by serogroups B and C.

Vaccine and Clinical Effectiveness

One meningococcal polysaccharide vaccine, quadrivalent A, C, Y, W-135, is available for use in the United States. Many studies have shown the immunogenicity, safety, and clinical efficacy of the group A and C polysaccharides. The group Y and W-135 polysaccharides have been shown to be safe and immunogenic in adults, but clinical protection has not been demonstrated in clinical trials. The duration of immunity conferred by the vaccine is unknown.

Indications

Routine vaccination of adults with meningococcal vaccine is not recommended because of the low risk of infection. Vaccination is recommended only for persons with specific high-risk conditions, including terminal complement component deficiency and anatomic or functional asplenia. Vaccinations may also be recommended for or required of travelers who visit areas recognized as having epidemic meningococcal disease. It may also be beneficial in the control of outbreaks caused by the vaccine serogroups in closed or semiclosed populations, such as college students.

Administration, Adverse Reactions, Precautions, Contraindications, and Revaccination

Meningococcal vaccine is given as a single dose (0.5 mL) intramuscularly. Adverse reactions are infrequent and mild, consisting principally of localized erythema at the injection site that lasts 1 to 2 days. The safety of meningococcal vaccine for pregnant women has not been established. Revaccination is not recommended.

Unresolved Issues

An effective serogroup B meningococcal vaccine is needed because this serogroup is a common cause of meningococcal disease in the United States. Current research is also focused on developing improved serogroup A and C vaccines.

Mumps

Mumps generally is a self-limited disease, but complications can occur when it develops in adults. Mumps orchitis can occur in as many as 38% of postpubertal boys and men with the disease, but it is usually unilateral and rarely results in sterility. Meningeal inflammation can occur in as many as 40% of cases. Nerve deafness occurs in approximately 1 in 15 000 cases.

The incidence of mumps in the United States dramatically decreased after the live mumps virus vaccine was introduced: in 1985 only 2982 cases were reported. There was a resurgence of mumps peaking at nearly 13 000 reported cases in 1987, but since then the incidence has decreased again to record low numbers. Although mumps vaccine was licensed in 1967, the Advisory Committee on Immunization Practices and the American Academy of Pediatrics did not recommend this vaccine for routine use until 1977 and 1982, respectively. This decision resulted in a cohort of teenagers and young adults who are insufficiently immunized. In 1991, 36% of reported mumps cases for which patient age was known occurred in those 15 years or older. Outbreaks in the mid-1980s occurred primarily among adolescents and young adults in high schools, colleges, and in occupational settings. Most of those affected had not been vaccinated, and the greatest risk for mumps occurred in states that had not implemented requirements for mumps vaccination for all students from kindergarten through grade 12. However, several outbreaks of mumps in widely vaccinated populations have been documented. The relative contributions of primary vaccine failure and waning immunity in these cases are unknown, but the former is thought to be the more important factor. The two-dose MMR vaccination schedule now recommended for children and selected adults should decrease the number of young adults who are susceptible to mumps and help prevent further outbreaks.

Vaccine and Clinical Effectiveness

Mumps vaccine is a live attenuated virus vaccine that is prepared in chick embryo cell culture. It is available as a monovalent (mumps only) vaccine, in combination with rubella vaccine, and in combination with measles and rubella as MMR vaccine. In most circumstances, MMR is the preferred vaccine.

A single dose of live attenuated mumps vaccine results in long-lasting protective levels of antibody in more than 90% of recipients. In epidemic situations, vaccine efficacy rates have ranged from 75% to 95%. The two-dose MMR schedule now recommended for children and selected adults is expected to provide protection to most persons who do not respond to their initial vaccination.

Indications

Mumps vaccine is indicated for all adults born after 1956 who lack documentation of immunization with live mumps vaccine on or after their first birthdays, physician-diagnosed mumps, or laboratory evidence of immunity. Special efforts should be made to ensure that all college and university students are immune to mumps because outbreaks have occurred in these settings.

Administration and Adverse Reactions

A single dose (0.5 mL) of reconstituted vaccine (preferably MMR) should be administered subcutaneously to susceptible adults. Parotitis after mumps vaccination has been reported rarely. Allergic reactions, including rash, pruritus, and purpura, have been temporally associated with vaccination, but they are uncommon, usually mild, and of brief duration. Encephalitis has been reported rarely after mumps vaccination. Vaccination of a person who already has naturally acquired or vaccine-induced immunity is not associated with adverse effects.

Precautions and Contraindications

Mumps vaccine should not be given for the 14 days before and several months after a person has received immune globulin, whole blood, or other antibody-containing blood products (*see* Table 1.6). Because of the theoretical risk for damage to the fetus, mumps vaccine should not be given to pregnant women. In women of childbearing age, adequate contraceptive measures should be ensured for 3 months after vaccination. In general, mumps vaccine should not be given to persons who are immunocompromised as a result of most immunodeficiency diseases, leukemia, lymphoma, or generalized malignancy, or to those who are immunosuppressed because of therapy with corticosteroids, alkylating agents, antimetabolites, or radiation. However, persons with leukemia who are in remission and have not received chemotherapy for at least 3 months and well persons with HIV may be vaccinated with MMR, if they are considered susceptible to mumps, and should be vaccinated if considered susceptible to measles.

Persons with a history of anaphylactic reactions (hives, swelling of the mouth and throat, difficulty in breathing, hypotension, or shock) after egg ingestion or receipt of neomycin should not be vaccinated. Persons with reactions that are not anaphylactic are not at increased risk and can be vaccinated.

Revaccination

Because immunity after a single dose of mumps vaccine is long lasting, no specific recommendation for mumps reimmunization exists. However, because MMR is generally used for the two-dose schedule for measles immunization, children and certain young adults are now receiving a second mumps immunization. This will benefit the approximately 5% of persons who do not respond to the first dose. The administration of mumps vaccine to persons who already have naturally acquired or vaccine-induced immunity is not associated with adverse effects.

Unresolved Issues

Because MMR has been given without incident to persons with HIV who are asymptomatic and to persons with leukemia in remission, it is recommended for such persons. The risks and benefits of this vaccine in relation to other conditions associated with immunocompromise are unknown.

Plague

The incidence of human plague has increased slowly in the United States, resulting in about 10 to 30 cases per year in the past two decades. The disease is maintained throughout the world in natural reservoirs by transmission of *Yersinia pestis* between many species of rodents and their fleas. Plague is found in the western United States and in parts of Asia, Africa, and South America. Carnivores, including cats and dogs, sometimes act as hosts. In rural and suburban areas in the western and southwestern states, human cases occur sporadically after rodent flea bites or after direct exposure to plague-infected animals. Exposure to infected domestic cats is of particular concern. The rural rodent disease can cause explosive urban epidemics among rats and their fleas, but urban plague is prevented by basic sanitation, urban rat control measures, and barriers between wild and urban rodent populations.

Vaccine and Clinical Effectiveness

Plague vaccine is an extract derived from formalin-inactivated *Y. pestis* grown in artificial media and preserved in 0.5% phenol. Vaccination produces passive hemagglutination antibody titers of 1:128 or greater in at least 90% of recipients, a level that is protective in animals. The efficacy of plague vaccine has not been directly measured in clinical trials. Field experience in Vietnam, where plague is endemic, showed protection against both disease and death among vaccinated military personnel. However, some cases of both the bubonic and primary pneumonic plagues have been reported in vaccinated persons. Therefore, antibiotics (for example, streptomycin or tetracycline) should be given to persons who have had a definite exposure, regardless of whether they have been vaccinated.

Indications

Veterinarians who treat small animals, especially cats, in regions where plague is endemic should be vaccinated because primary pneumonic plague has been transmitted by aerosols from sick cats. Laboratory workers, ecologists, and others working directly with *Y. pestis* or wild rodents in endemic regions should be considered for plague vaccination. Clinical microbiology laboratory workers, health care workers, and most travelers to plague-endemic areas do not need to be vaccinated. Vaccination against plague is not recommended for persons living in or traveling to plague-endemic areas unless substantial exposure to plague-infected rodents is anticipated.

Administration, Adverse Reactions, Precautions, and Contraindications

A primary series of plague vaccination consists of three intramuscular doses, the first dose (1.0 mL) followed by two smaller doses (0.2 mL each) given at 1 and at 3 to 6 months. Approximately 10% of persons receiving a primary series experience local pain or swelling, malaise, headache, fever, or mild adenopathy. More severe reactions can occur with revaccination and in persons who are allergic to components of the vaccine. Rare cases of urticaria, asthma, and sterile abscess have been reported. Persons who are allergic to beef protein, soya, casein, or phenol should not be given plague vaccine.

Revaccination

If exposure to *Y. pestis* is expected to continue, two booster doses (0.2 mL each) should be given at 6-month intervals. Booster doses (0.2 mL each) may then be given at 1- or 2-year intervals. Persons who have had serious reactions to previous doses of plague vaccine should not be revaccinated.

Pneumococcal Infections

The annual burden of invasive pneumococcal disease in the United States is approximately 500 000 cases of pneumonia; 50 000 cases of sepsis; and 3000 cases of meningitis. Pneumococcal infections cause approximately 40 000 deaths each year. The pneumococcus (*Streptococcus pneumoniae*) causes about one third of all adult pneumonias and many cases of acute bacterial bronchitis. Most of these illnesses are nonbacteremic infections that cause considerable morbidity but few deaths and are difficult to confirm microbiologically. The overall case-fatality rate in treated pneumonia patients is 5% to 8%. Pneumococci are also an under-recognized but important cause of nosocomial pneumonia.

The case-fatality rate of pneumococcal bacteremia is approximately 20%. Race and age are important risk factors. Alaskan natives have very high rates of invasive pneumococcal disease. Black adults have about three to five times higher incidence rates of pneumococcal bacteremia than do comparably aged white persons. In persons 65 years and older, the annual incidence of pneumococcal bacteremia is more than 50 cases per 100 000 persons. In most communities, pneumococcal infections continue to be the leading cause of adult community-acquired pneumonia requiring hospitalization. The incidence of pneumococcal disease and the case-fatality rate increase with underlying medical conditions such as chronic cardiac and pulmonary disease, hepatic and renal failure, alcoholism, anatomic and functional asplenia, multiple myeloma, and Hodgkin disease. The case-fatality rate of treated bacteremic disease is 15% to 25%, but, among patients with underlying medical conditions, it increases to 30% or more. In elderly patients with pneumococcal bacteremia, the mortality rate can be as high as 60%. In patients with pneumococcal meningitis, the overall mortality rate is 20% but increases to 65% in patients older than 70 years. Human immunodeficiency virus infection is an important risk factor for pneumococcal infection, with an annual attack rate as high as 1%. The mortality rates for pneumococcal infections have not decreased substantially in recent decades, despite the prompt use of appropriate antimicrobial therapy and intensive care. Most deaths occur in patients who are irreversibly injured early in the course of their infections.

Resistance of *S. pneumoniae* to penicillin is rapidly increasing worldwide; in several European countries, about one quarter of clinical isolates of pneumococci are resistant to penicillin. Many of these penicillin-resistant isolates are also resistant to commonly used anti-pneumococcal antibiotics such as erythromycin, chloramphenicol, and cotrimoxazole. Although most pneumococcal isolates from the United States continue to be sensitive to penicillin and to other antimicrobial drugs, surveillance studies show an increasing proportion of antimicrobial-resistant strains of *S. pneumoniae*. This ominous trend underscores the importance of ensuring that persons at risk for acquiring severe pneumococcal infections are immunized.

Vaccine

The pneumococcal vaccine used since 1983 contains the capsular polysaccharides of the 23 pneumococcal types responsible for 85% to 90% of bacteremia infections. This vaccine replaced a 14-valent formulation licensed in 1977. Pneumococcal capsular polysaccharide antigens induce type-specific antibodies that enhance the opsonization, phagocytosis, and killing of pneumococci by leukocytes and fixed phagocytic cells. During untreated pneumococcal infection, the development of detectable type-specific antibody after 7 to 10 days coincides with the classic "crisis" that was characterized by termination of bacteremia, resolution of clinical illness, and protection against reinfection with the same type. Many of the conditions associated with an increased incidence of pneumococcal infections or high case-fatality rates are characterized by a decreased antibody response or impaired phagocytic clearance of pneumococcal organisms.

The 23-valent vaccine contains 25 µg of each capsular polysaccharide antigen (14-valent vaccine contained 50 µg of each antigen). After vaccination with 14-valent or 23-valent vaccine, a twofold or greater increase in antibody titer to each antigen develops in 80% or more of healthy young adults. Antibody levels decrease in the next 6 to 12 months, but in most persons high levels are maintained for at least 7 to 10 years. Among elderly subjects, antibody levels appear to decrease more rapidly than in young adults and may decline to levels not considered protective after 6 or more years.

Pneumococcal vaccination increases antibody levels in elderly patients and in those with insulin-requiring diabetes mellitus, chronic obstructive pulmonary disease, and alcoholic cirrhosis. In these persons, total antibody levels and responses to individual antigens may be lower than in healthy young adults, but they are still considered adequate for protection. Antibody responses are also excellent in patients with sickle cell disease or in those who have had splenectomy. In Hodgkin disease, pneumococcal vaccination is effective if given before splenectomy, radiation, or chemotherapy; however, after treatment has begun, these patients respond less well, and preexisting antibodies may be expected to decrease. In patients with leukemia, lymphoma, multiple myeloma, and HIV infection, the antibody response to pneumococcal vaccination is suboptimal. In hemodialysis patients, renal transplant recipients, and those with the nephrotic syndrome, the initial antibody response is lower and/or antibody levels decrease more rapidly than in healthy persons.

Clinical Effectiveness

In assessing vaccine efficacy, recognize that the vaccine is composed of 23 individual polysaccharide vaccines. The recipient's immune response may not be uniform to each component, and each serotype vaccine has its own failure rate. Thus, it is not unexpected that in patients exposed to multiple serotypes of *S. pneumoniae,* the protective efficacy of the 23-valent vaccine is incomplete.

In earlier randomized, controlled trials among United States military recruits, South African gold miners, and New Guinea highlanders, a pneumococcal vaccine was shown to be very protective against pneumococcal pneumonia and bacteremia in healthy young adults in settings with high rates of pneumococcal disease. In several studies of older, high-risk patients, vaccine efficacy was less consistent. Trials to evaluate the effectiveness of pneumococcal vaccine are difficult because the incidence of pneumococcal disease is low and consequently large study populations are required. In the United States, three randomized, placebo-controlled trials in older adults did not show pneumococcal vaccine to be protective. In a prepaid medical plan in San Francisco, a clinical trial among 13 600 adults 45 years or older showed no reduction in the total incidence of pneumonia in those who received vaccine. A small clinical trial in a chronic disease hospital yielded similar results. In a Veterans Administration multicenter clinical trial that randomized 2295 high-risk patients, no difference in the frequency of non-bacteremic pneumococcal pneumonia or bronchitis in vaccine recipients was found compared with control patients. Antibody responses to vaccination in some patients were suboptimal. In this trial, cases of bacteremia were too few to measure vaccine efficacy. Finally, in one case-control study that compared rates of vaccination in patients with and without pneumococcal bacteremia, no vaccine efficacy was shown. This last study had relatively few patients, and vaccine recipients tended to be older and more immunocompromised.

In contrast to these reports, several case-control studies showed pneumococcal vaccination to be effective. In one study of 122 patients with bacteremia and 244 matched controls, pneumococcal vaccine was 70% protective in immunocompetent elderly patients. A second, larger case-control study reported that 543 patients with invasive pneumococcal infections received vaccine significantly less frequently than did 543 matched noninfected controls (13% compared with 23%). The most comprehensive case-control study involved 1054 patients with serious pneumococcal disease who met an indication for pneumococcal vaccine and an equal number of hospital-based controls matched according to age, underlying disease, and site of hospitalization. The aggregate protective efficacy of the vaccine was 56%; protective efficacy was higher in younger, immunocompetent patients. As part of this study, pneumococcal isolates were collected; there were 170 pairs of case-patients and controls in which the case-patient was infected with a pneumococcal serotype not included in the 23- valent vaccine. Vaccine efficacy in this group was nil, which corroborated evidence that the vaccine was effective only against serotypes represented in the vaccine.

TABLE 8.11.   Pneumococcal Vaccine Coverage and Prevalence of High-Risk Conditions

Age Group	Persons at High Risk			Persons at High Risk Who Received Pneumococcal Vaccine
	Whites	Nonwhites	Total	
y	◄───────────		% ─────────────►	
50–64	30.6	38.2	31.5	8.4
>64	46.8	53.3	47.4	15.4

Source: Centers for Disease Control and Prevention.

After assessing the results of these studies, pneumococcal vaccine appears to be safe. The vaccine effectively reduces the incidence of pneumococcal bacteremia and pneumonia among younger patients, in whom rates of pneumococcal disease are high. Pneumococcal vaccination also appears to be effective in reducing the incidence of pneumococcal bacteremia among older, high-risk patients who have good antibody responses to vaccination. The efficacy of pneumococcal vaccine, as measured in case-control studies, is significantly decreased in immunosuppressed patients. No data on pneumococcal vaccine efficacy in patients with HIV infection exist.

Indications

Pneumococcal vaccine is indicated for adult patients with underlying conditions that are associated with increased susceptibility to infection or increased risk for serious disease and its complications.

Table 8.11 summarizes information from the 1985 U.S. Immunization Survey and compares the percentage of persons at high risk to the fraction immunized with pneumococcal vaccine. About one third of persons ages 50 to 64 years have at least one medical condition that would permit receipt of pneumococcal vaccine, yet, in 1985, only 8.4% of persons at high risk received pneumococcal vaccine. In persons older than 64 years, about one half had at least one high-risk condition, yet only 15% received pneumococcal vaccine. More recent data from the 1991 National Health Interview Survey show that only about 20% of persons 65 years or older had ever received a dose of pneumococcal vaccine. These data, despite their limitations, suggest that many persons considered to be at risk for pneumococcal infection have not received pneumococcal vaccine.

High-risk patients include those with chronic cardiac and pulmonary disease (especially congestive heart failure, recurrent bronchitis, or chronic obstructive lung disease), anatomic or functional asplenia, chronic liver disease, alcoholism, and diabetes mellitus. Patients with chronic renal failure, Hodgkin disease, chronic lymphatic leukemia, multiple myeloma, and those receiving hemodialysis, chemotherapy for carcinoma, or organ transplants should also be vaccinated, but they may have diminished antibody responses and should be told so.

Despite the lack of evidence showing efficacy, persons with HIV infection should be vaccinated as soon as possible, on the grounds of clinical prudence, because they are at high risk for acquiring pneumococcal disease, and their antibody response is better in the earlier phases of HIV infection. Whenever possible, pneumococcal vaccine should be given in advance of elective splenectomy or planned chemotherapy to maximize the antibody response.

The Task Force strongly recommends that the 50th birthday be used as a special date to review overall immunization status; to give a tetanus-diphtheria booster if indicated; and to determine specifically whether the patient should receive a dose of pneumococcal vaccine and begin annual influenza immunization. Between 30% and 40% of persons 50 to 65 years old have high-risk conditions that define them as candidates for pneumococcal vaccine. The prevalence of these conditions is likely to be even higher among those regularly seeking medical care. Thus, physicians should be aggressive in identifying such conditions in their patients and in providing vaccine. For healthy adults (those without risk factors), universal immunization with pneumococcal vaccine should be provided at age 65 years. This is also an appropriate time to consider revaccinating those with high-risk conditions who received their first immunization more than 6 years earlier.

Administration

Pneumococcal vaccine should be given as a single intramuscular or subcutaneous dose (0.5 mL). Hospital discharge is a convenient time to determine the need for pneumococcal vaccine because approximately two thirds of all patients who are hospitalized with serious pneumococcal infections were discharged from the hospital within the previous 5 years. Annual influenza vaccination should serve as a reminder to review the status of pneumococcal vaccination.

The indications for pneumococcal and influenza vaccines are similar, and administration of influenza vaccine should automatically trigger a review of whether the patient has ever received pneumococcal vaccine. Both pneumococcal and influenza vaccines can be given simultaneously but at different sites, with no decrease in the antibody responses nor increase in adverse reactions. The cost of both pneumococcal and influenza vaccines and their administration is partially reimbursed by Medicare.

Adverse Reactions, Precautions and Contraindications

Pneumococcal vaccine is safe. Minor local side effects such as pain or redness are common after pneumococcal vaccination, occurring in as many as 50% of persons given the vaccine. More severe allergic or systemic reactions such as fever or rash are rare, occurring in fewer than 1% of recipients. Local Arthus-like reactions have sometimes been reported after early second doses of 14-valent vaccine but are very infrequent after revaccination with the current 23-valent vaccine and are very rare if 6 or more years have elapsed since the first pneumococcal vaccination. No neurologic disorders, such as the Guillain-Barré syndrome, have been linked to pneumococcal vaccine. Adverse consequences to the fetus have not been reported among women vaccinated during pregnancy. Pregnant women with high-risk conditions such as cardiac, pulmonary, or sickle cell disease may be vaccinated, although it is preferable to vaccinate after the first trimester or before pregnancy.

Revaccination

Revaccination with 23-valent vaccine is recommended for all persons who received 14-valent pneumococcal vaccine if they are at highest risk of serious or fatal pneumococcal infection (for example, patients with surgical or functional asplenia). Revaccination is also recommended for adults at highest risk who received the 23-valent vaccine 6 or more years previously and for those shown to have rapid decreases in pneumococcal antibody levels (for example, patients with the nephrotic syndrome, renal failure, or transplant recipients). In these patients, adverse reactions after revaccination have not been a problem. Although immunologic data are lacking, reimmunization at age 65 years should be strongly considered for those with high-risk conditions who received their first immunization more than 6 years earlier. A recommendation for routine revaccination with pneumococcal vaccine in healthy elderly persons cannot be made.

Unresolved Issues

The most important unresolved issue for pneumococcal vaccine is the need to improve its immunogenicity and protective efficacy. The lack of equivalent protective efficacy for each of the 23 capsular polysaccharide antigens is a related problem. A protein-conjugate vaccine holds promise of being more uniformly immunogenic. The optimal time for initial vaccination and the indications for revaccination must be determined. Serologic studies of antibody decay in a wide age range are urgently needed. Finally, better systems for delivering pneumococcal vaccine to high-risk persons are needed; efforts to date have reached only 10% to 20% of patients who should be vaccinated.

Poliomyelitis

The individual risk for acquiring paralytic poliomyelitis in the United States is small. No indigenous cases of wild-type poliovirus-caused disease have occurred here since 1979. The World Health Organization is involved in a worldwide effort to eradicate poliomyelitis. Great success has followed this initiative in the western hemisphere, where the last proven case of poliomyelitis due to wild-type virus transmission occurred in Peru in August 1991. However, paralytic poliomyelitis could reappear if high levels of immunity in the general population are not maintained by immunizing children routinely, or if wild-type poliovirus is introduced into populations that have become susceptible because of low rates of polio vaccination.

Vaccine and Clinical Effectiveness

Two types of poliovirus vaccine are available in the United States: oral polio vaccine and an enhanced-potency inactivated polio vaccine. Both are trivalent vaccines that contain antigens of the three poliovirus types (I, II, and III).

A primary series with either vaccine produces immunity to all three poliovirus types in more than 95% of recipients. Immunity in most persons is probably lifelong.

Indications

Routine polio vaccination of adults living in the United States who have not had a primary series as children is not necessary. However, previously unvaccinated adults who are at increased risk for exposure to wild-type polioviruses because of foreign travel or work as health care providers should receive primary series of polio vaccine. Enhanced-potency inactivated polio vaccine is preferred because the risk for oral polio vaccine-associated paralysis is slightly higher in adults than in children. However, if protection is needed in fewer than 4 weeks, a single dose of oral polio vaccine or enhanced-potency inactivated polio vaccine is recommended. Travelers who previously received less than a full primary course of oral or inactivated polio vaccine should receive the remaining required doses of either vaccine, regardless of the interval since the last dose. Travelers who previously completed a primary series of either oral or inactivated polio vaccine should receive a single booster dose of oral polio vaccine or enhanced-potency inactivated polio vaccine.

Administration

A primary series for oral polio vaccine consists of three doses: two doses given 6 to 8 weeks apart and a third dose given at least 6 weeks, and customarily 8 to 12 months, after the second dose. A primary series for enhanced-potency inactivated polio vaccine consists of three doses (0.5 mL each) given subcutaneously: two doses given 4 to 8 weeks apart and a third dose given at least 4 weeks, and preferably 6 to 12 months, after the second.

For persons who have received only part of a primary series of polio vaccine, the series can be completed with enhanced-potency inactivated polio vaccine or oral polio vaccine. If oral polio vaccine was used initially, three doses of a mixed enhanced-potency inactivated polio vaccine and oral polio vaccine schedule will complete the primary series. If inactivated polio vaccine was used for the earlier doses, the primary series should include four doses and can be completed with either oral polio vaccine or enhanced-potency inactivated polio vaccine.

Adverse Reactions

Oral Polio Vaccine: Administration of oral polio vaccine rarely has been associated with paralysis in vaccine recipients and their contacts. The risks of vaccine-associated paralytic poliomyelitis are small: among first-dose recipients, approximately 1 case per 1.2 million first doses distributed; among contacts of first-dose recipients, approximately 1 case per 1 million first doses distributed. The overall risk is 1 case per 520 000 first doses distributed. The risks for vaccine-associated poliomyelitis after subsequent doses of vaccine are further reduced. Recipients and their contacts should be informed of these risks.

Enhanced-Potency Inactivated Polio Vaccine: No serious adverse effects to inactivated polio vaccines have been documented. Because the enhanced-potency inactivated polio vaccine may contain trace amounts of streptomycin, neomycin, or polymyxin B, hypersensitivity reactions can occur in persons sensitive to these antibiotics. Persons who experience anaphylactic reactions after receiving neomycin should not receive the inactivated vaccine. Persons with reactions to neomycin that are not anaphylactic in nature are not at increased risk and can be vaccinated.

Precautions and Contraindications

Oral Polio Vaccine: Oral polio vaccine should not be given to persons who are definitely or possibly immunocompromised as a result of immunodeficiency diseases (including HIV infection), leukemia, lymphoma, or generalized malignancy, or immunosuppressed because of therapy with corticosteroids, alkylating drugs, antimetabolites, or radiation. If polio immunization is indicated, enhanced-potency inactivated polio vaccine should be used; some protection may result from its administration. The same guidelines apply to household contacts of oral polio vaccine recipients who are immunocompromised for any reason.

Adults who are not adequately immunized against poliomyelitis have a very small risk for developing vaccine-associated poliomyelitis when children in the household are given oral polio vaccine. Nonetheless, because of the overriding importance of prompt and complete immunization of children, and the extreme rarity of oral polio vaccine-associated disease in contacts, the standard practice is administration of oral polio vaccine to children regardless of the polio vaccination status of adult household contacts. The responsible adult should be informed of the small risk involved and the precautions to be taken, such as hand washing after changing diapers. An acceptable alternative, if there is strong assurance that complete immunization of the child will not be jeopardized or unduly delayed, is administration of at least two doses of enhanced-potency inactivated polio vaccine to previously unimmunized adults before giving oral polio vaccine to the child.

Enhanced-Potency Inactivated Vaccine: Although no convincing evidence of adverse effects of inactivated polio vaccine in pregnant women or developing fetuses exists, it is prudent on theoretical grounds to avoid vaccination during pregnancy. However, if immediate protection against poliomyelitis is needed, a single dose of either oral polio vaccine or enhanced-potency inactivated polio vaccine should be given. If time permits, two doses of enhanced-potency inactivated polio vaccine are preferred.

Revaccination

For persons who have completed a primary series of oral polio vaccine or inactivated polio vaccine, the only indication for revaccination is a one-time booster dose for travelers to foreign countries where poliomyelitis is endemic. This ensures an adequate immune response to each of the three poliovirus types.

Unresolved Issues

The major controversy surrounding polio immunization is whether routine use of enhanced-potency inactivated polio vaccine should supplant use of oral polio vaccine in children to prevent the 5 to 10 cases of paralytic poliomyelitis associated with oral polio vaccination each year. The Institute of Medicine re-examined this question and recommends continuing use of oral polio vaccine. When enhanced-potency inactivated polio vaccine is licensed for use with DTP vaccine, this recommendation may change

Rabies

Rabies virus is maintained in many carnivorous species. Human infection usually results from a bite inoculation with virus-laden saliva. Rarely have humans become infected through contamination of scratches, abrasions, open cuts, wounds, or mucous membranes with saliva or other rabies virus-infected materials. Some cases have been attributed to aerosol transmission in rabies research laboratories (two cases) or to bat-infested caves (two cases), presumably through infection of the respiratory tract and subsequent spread from this site. Corneas harvested from donors with encephalitis of unknown cause resulted in five cases of fatal rabies in corneal transplant recipients. These episodes are the only documented instances of human-to-human transmission.

After inoculation, the virus replicates locally and spreads through peripheral nerves to the central nervous system, where it causes encephalitis. The initial site of virus inoculation affects the likelihood of developing clinical rabies and the length of the incubation period. For example, if the virus is introduced by a severe bite on the face, the risk for developing rabies is approximately 60%; if the bite is on the hand or arm, the risk decreases to 15% to 40%; if it is on the leg, the risk is only 3% to 10%. Typically, rabies occurring after a bite on the face, arm, or hand has a shorter incubation period (approximately 40 days), whereas longer incubation periods (50 days or more) have been reported when the virus was inoculated at other body sites.

Clinical rabies usually begins with nonspecific constitutional symptoms. Within 1 week, neurologic dysfunction becomes apparent and can result in one of two clinical manifestations: the more common furious form (hydrophobia, aerophobia, bizarre behavior, seizures, nuchal rigidity, agitation) or the less common paralytic form. Rabies should be considered in any patient with rapidly progressive encephalitis of unknown cause. Only three instances of recovery from rabies have been reported, and none since 1977. Despite these recoveries, rabies must be regarded as a fatal disease, and the emphasis should be on prevention rather than treatment.

Prevention of rabies depends on adequate immunization. In persons who have had an exposure or potential exposure to rabies, human rabies immune globulin (HRIG) is given to provide protective antibody immediately. At the same time, vaccination is begun to ensure long-term protection. For persons with an ongoing risk of rabies exposure, pre-exposure prophylaxis with sons with an ongoing risk of rabies exposure, pre-exposure prophylaxis with vaccine is recommended.

Vaccine

The rabies vaccine used in the United States since 1982 is human diploid cell rabies vaccine (HDCV). It is considerably more potent and has a much lower risk for adverse effects than the duck embryo vaccine used from 1957 to 1982. The vaccine virus is inactivated with beta-propriolactone. The rabies vaccines used in many developing countries contain inactivated virus grown in animal neural tissue. These vaccines have a much higher risk for adverse effects and also may be less potent.

In 1988, a second rabies vaccine, adsorbed (RVA), was licensed for use in the United States. It is grown in a diploid cell line of fetal rhesus lung and is produced by the Biologics Products Program, Michigan Department of Public Health.

Human Rabies Immune Globulin

Rabies immune globulin is obtained from the plasma of hyperimmunized human donors. Its antirabies neutralizing antibody content is standardized to contain 150 international units (IU) per milliliter, and is available in 2-mL (300 IU) and 10-mL (1500 IU) vials.

Clinical Effectiveness

Each year approximately 18 000 persons receive antirabies postexposure prophylaxis in the United States, although most have not had a significant rabies exposure. Rabies has not developed in anyone exposed to rabies in the United States who had received the recommended intramuscular schedule of HDCV and HRIG. In addition, field trials in countries where rabies is endemic have shown that postexposure prophylaxis with HDCV and HRIG is very effective.

Rabies vaccine, adsorbed, induces an antirabies neutralizing antibody response comparable to that achieved with HDCV after intramuscular immunization. However, RVA has not been evaluated or approved for intradermal administration.

Indications

Pre-exposure prophylaxis with HDCV should be offered to persons continually at risk for contact with rabies virus. These persons include veterinarians and their staff, animal handlers, certain laboratory and wildlife workers, and those spending prolonged time in countries where rabies is endemic. In particular, persons whose professional or recreational activities place them in frequent contact with potentially rabid dogs, cats, foxes, raccoons, skunks, bats, or other species at risk for having rabies should be considered for pre-exposure prophylaxis. A history of pre-exposure prophylaxis does not eliminate the need for postexposure prophylaxis; it only simplifies the postexposure program. Table 8.12 outlines the guidelines for pre-exposure prophylaxis.

Postexposure prophylaxis is indicated whenever a possible rabies exposure has occurred. In the United States and other parts of the developed world, successful animal vaccination programs have reduced the occurrence of rabies among domestic dogs and cats and, thus, their importance as a source of human rabies. For example, in 1946 more than 8000 cases of dog rabies were identified in the United States; 40 years later only approximately 150 cases were known. However, in other areas of the world, including most of Asia and all of Africa and Latin America, dogs are still the primary source of human rabies. Five of the 12 rabies deaths that occurred in American citizens between 1980 and 1992 were caused by exposure to rabid dogs in other countries. In the United States, more than 85% of animal rabies occurs in nondomesticated species, especially bats, skunks, foxes, and raccoons. Bats have accounted for five of the seven indigenously acquired human rabies cases reported from 1980 through 1991. Because bat bites can be very small (and even missed on physical examination), postexposure treatment for persons who have had physical contact with a bat is prudent when a bite or mucous membrane exposure cannot be excluded. Animals that are rarely infected with rabies virus include rodents (squirrels, hamsters, ferrets, guinea pigs, gerbils, chipmunks, rats, and mice) and lagomorphs (rabbits and hares). Most courses of postexposure prophylaxis given in the United States are given after dog and cat bites. Table 8.13 provides general guidelines for postexposure prophylaxis.

Administration

Pre-exposure Prophylaxis: The intramuscular route of administration is preferred. Three injections (1 mL each) of HDCV should be given intramuscularly in the deltoid, one each on days, 0, 7, and 28. The same schedule is followed when RVA is used. Antibody testing after vaccination should be considered. As outlined in Table 8.12, persons with continual high-level exposure to rabies should have their antibody titers measured every 6 months, with booster injections (1 mL) given as often as needed. Persons with less intensive exposure (for example, veterinarians and spelunkers) should be revaccinated (1 mL) every 2 years, or have their antibody titers checked and receive booster injections whenever rabies neutralizing antibody titers become

TABLE 8.12. Indications for Pre-exposure Prophylaxis for Rabies

Risk Category	Nature of Risk	Typical Populations	Need for Pre-exposure Rabies Prophylaxis*	
			Primary Vaccination	Booster Vaccination
Continuous	Virus present continually, often in high concentrations; aerosol, mucous membrane, bite, or nonbite exposure possible; specific exposures may go unrecognized	Rabies research laboratory workers; rabies biologics production workers	Yes	Yes[†]
Frequent	Exposure usually episodic, with source recognized, but exposure may be unrecognized; aerosol, mucous membrane, bite, or nonbite exposure	Rabies diagnostic laboratory workers; spelunkers; veterinarians; animal control and wildlife workers in rabies-epizootic areas	Yes	Yes[‡]
Infrequent	Exposure nearly always episodic with source recognized; mucous membrane, bite, or nonbite exposure	Veterinarians and animal control and wildlife workers in areas of low rabies endemicity; foreign travelers to rabies-epizootic areas; veterinary students	Yes	No
Rare	Exposure always episodic; mucous membrane or bite with source known	United States population at large, including persons in rabies-epizootic areas	No	No

* Primary vaccination for pre-exposure rabies prophylaxis consists of three doses (1 mL each) intramuscularly on days 0, 7, and 28. Either human diploid cell vaccine (HDVC) or rabies vaccine, adsorbed (RVA), can be used. Alternatively, three doses of HDCV (but not RVA) can be given intradermally, 0.1 mL on days 0, 7, and 28. Booster vaccination consists of a single dose of HDCV or RVA given intramuscularly (1 mL) or intradermally (0.1 mL of HDCV but not RVA). See text for details.

[†] Rabies antibody levels should be measured every 6 months and booster doses of vaccine given when rabies-neutralizing antibody levels decrease to inadequate levels (0.5 Iu/mL serum).

[‡] Booster vaccination or serologic testing every 2 years.

Source: Modified from MMWR. 1991;40(RR-3):1–19.

TABLE 8.13. Indications for Postexposure Prophylaxis for Rabies*

Animal	Condition of Animal at Time of Attack	Treatment of Exposed Person
Dog, cat	Healthy and available for 10 days of observation Rabid or suspected rabid Unknown (escaped)	None unless animal develops rabies Rabies vaccine and HRIG Consult public health officials; if treatment is indicated, give rabies vaccine and HRIG
Skunk, bat, fox, coyote, raccoon, bobcat, and other carnivores	Regard as rabid unless proved negative by laboratory test	Rabies vaccine and HRIG
Livestock, rodents, rabbits, hares	Consider individually	Consult public health officials. Bites of squirrels, hamsters, guinea pigs, gerbils, ferrets, chipmunks, rats, mice, or other rodents, rabbits, and hares almost never require antirabies prophylaxis

* Rabies vaccines include human diploid cell vaccine (HDCV) and rabies vaccine, adsorbed (RVA). HRIG = human rabies immune globulin. For persons who previously received pre-exposure rabies prophylaxis, cleansing of the wound, and two doses of rabies vaccine (1 mL intramuscularly [IM], *not* intradermally [ID], on days 0 and 3) are sufficient. For persons who previously have not received pre-exposure prophylaxis, five doses of rabies vaccine (1 mL IM, *not* ID, on days 0, 3, 7, 14, and 28) and one dose of HRIG 920 IU/kg IM, on day 0, are necessary. See text for details.
Source: Modified from MMWR. 1991;40(RR–3):1–19.

inadequate (0.5 IU/mL serum).

Several state health department laboratories provide rabies antibody testing (including New York, Maryland, and California). In addition, testing can be obtained from the Department of Veterinary Diagnostics, College of Veterinary Medicine, Kansas State University, Manhattan, KS 66506-5600; 913-532-5650.

An alternative, less costly approach to pre-exposure prophylaxis uses three 0.1-mL doses of HDCV (but not RVA) administered intradermally. The vaccine is supplied in single-dose syringes containing lyophilized vaccine that is reconstituted immediately before use. Intradermal vaccination of immunocompetent persons produces seroconversion rates that are somewhat lower than those obtained with intramuscular administration. Mean antibody titers are also slightly lower and duration of immunity may be shorter. Antibody levels should be confirmed 2 to 4 weeks after the third dose of vaccine. Poor response to intradermal vaccination has been observed in persons receiving chloroquine for malaria prophylaxis.

Postexposure Prophylaxis: The indications for postexposure prophylaxis are given in Table 8.13. The first step is immediate cleansing of the wound with soap and water (Table 8.14). In persons with no previous history of antirabies immunization, HRIG (20 IU/kg) must be administered immediately. As much as one half of the dose should be given in and around the area of the wound (when anatomically feasible), with the rest administered intramuscularly. Five doses (1.0 mL each) of HDCV (or RVA) are administered intramuscularly in the deltoid, one dose each on days 0, 3, 7, 14, and 28. The intradermal dose (0.1 mL) and route should not be used for postexposure prophylaxis. Because HRIG can partially suppress the antibody response to the vaccine, no more than the recommended dose of HRIG should be given. Rabies immune globulin and rabies vaccine should not be administered in the same syringe or at the same anatomic site.

Persons who received complete and up-to-date pre-exposure immunization against rabies should have their wounds cleaned, but they do not require HRIG. Two booster doses (1.0 mL each) of HDCV (or RVA) should be given intramuscularly on days 0 and 3.

Appropriate tetanus prophylaxis should be given to all persons evaluated for a rabies exposure. Use of modified live rabies vaccine for animals was discontinued in the United States in 1991. Persons who are inadvertently exposed (from a needle-stick injury, for example) when administering inactivated rabies vaccine to animals are at no risk for contracting rabies.

TABLE 8.14.   Rabies Postexposure Prophylaxis Schedule*

Vaccination Status	Treatment	Regimen[†]
Not previously vaccinated	Local wound cleansing	All postexposure treatment should begin with immediate thorough cleansing of all wounds with soap and water.
	HRIG	20 IU/kg body weight. If anatomically feasible, up to one half of the dose should be infiltrated around the wound(s) and the rest should be administered IM in the gluteal area. HRIG should not be administered in the same syringe or into the same anatomic site as vaccine. Because HRIG may partially suppress active production of antibody, no more than the recommended dose should be given.
	Vaccine	HDCV or RVA, 1 mL IM (deltoid area, one each on days 0, 3, 7, 14, and 28)[‡]
Previously vaccinated[§]	Local wound cleansing	All postexposure treatment should begin with immediate thorough cleansing of all wounds with soap and water.
	HRIG	HRIG should not be administered.
	Vaccine	HDCV or RVA, 1 mL IM (deltoid area, one each on days 0 and 3)[‡]

* IM = intramuscular; HRIG = human rabies immune globulin; HDCV = human diploid cell vaccine; RVA = rabies vaccine, adsorbed
[†] These regimens are applicable for all age groups, including children. Appropriate tetanus prophylaxis also should be given.
[‡] The deltoid area is the only acceptable site of vaccination for adults and older children. For younger children, the outer thigh may be used. Vaccine should never be administered in the gluteal area.
[§] Any person with a history of pre-exposure vaccination with HDCV or RVA; previous postexposure prophylaxis with HDCV or RVA; or previous vaccination with any other type of rabies vaccine and a documented history of antibody response to the previous vaccination.

Adverse Reactions

Adverse reactions to HDCV and RVA occur less frequently than they did with previous rabies vaccines. Mild local reactions at the injection site develop in 25% to 50% of vaccine recipients. As many as 20% have mild headache, nausea, abdominal pain, myalgias, and dizziness. After booster injections of HDCV, an immune complex-like syndrome, characterized by urticaria and sometimes fever, malaise, arthralgias, arthritis, nausea, and vomiting, develops in approximately 6% of recipients. These symptoms appear 2 to 21 days after booster vaccination and have been associated with beta-propiolactone-altered human serum in HDCV. They are less common when RVA is used. Serious reactions such as anaphylaxis or the Guillain-Barré syndrome are rare.

Local pain and low-grade fever can occur after administration of HRIG. More serious reactions such as anaphylaxis are rare and are seen primarily in persons with IgA deficiency. No evidence exists that hepatitis B and C viruses, HIV, or other viruses have been transmitted by HRIG commercially available in the United States.

Precautions and Contraindications

Immunosuppression of any kind, including that caused by high-dose corticosteroids, can interfere with the antibody response to rabies vaccination. Immunosuppressive therapy should be avoided, if possible, during pre-exposure and postexposure prophylaxis. If this cannot be done, consideration should be given to administering additional doses of HDCV or measuring the antibody response and providing additional doses if needed.

No information exists to suggest that administration of HDCV, RVA, or HRIG during pregnancy causes fetal damage. Given the consequences of rabies exposure, pregnancy should not be considered a contraindication to postexposure prophylaxis. If it is believed that exposure to rabies virus is likely to occur, pre-exposure prophylaxis should be administered before pregnancy if possible.

The concurrent administration of chloroquine phosphate and other antimalarial agents for malaria chemoprophylaxis may interfere with the antibody response to intradermally administered HDCV. Thus, the administration of the three-dose intradermal series must be completed before antimalarial prophylaxis is begun. If this is not possible, the intramuscular schedule should be used.

Unresolved Issues

Because of its lower volume and cost, it would be useful to determine whether intradermal vaccination can reliably provide postexposure prophylaxis in underdeveloped areas of the world.

Rubella

Rubella infection that occurs in early pregnancy, especially in the first trimester, may result in abortion, miscarriage, stillbirth, or other congenital abnormalities. In fact, the congenital rubella syndrome can occur in as many as 80% of infected fetuses. Thus, preventing fetal infection and consequent congenital rubella syndrome is the primary objective of rubella immunization.

Rubella was once a common childhood disease. Universal immunization of children has interrupted its transmission throughout most of the United States. The reported occurrence of rubella decreased steadily from more than 57 000 cases in 1969, the year rubella vaccine was licensed, to 225 cases in 1988. Rubella incidence increased five to six times from 1990 to 1991, primarily in teenagers and young adults, but then returned to record low levels in 1992 and 1993. In 1990 and 1991, 41% and 45%, respectively, of cases of known age occurred in those 15 years and older. From 1984 through 1989, an annual average of 5.5 cases of the congenital rubella syndrome were reported in the United States. However, concomitant with the increase in rubella cases was a resurgence of the congenital rubella syndrome, with a marked increase in cases reported in 1990 and 1991. Of the 75 confirmed cases of the congenital rubella syndrome reported from 1986 through 1991, 48% might have been prevented by postpartum vaccination of susceptible women. An estimated 6% to 11% of young adults remain susceptible to rubella, and limited outbreaks continue to be reported in colleges, places of employment (notably hospitals), and in largely unvaccinated populations such as the Amish.

Vaccination of young children has prevented widespread epidemics of rubella and the congenital rubella syndrome and eventually should eliminate this syndrome as vaccinated cohorts reach childbearing age. However, increased efforts to ensure that all women of childbearing age are vaccinated can hasten the elimination of rubella and the congenital rubella syndrome in the United States.

Vaccine and Clinical Effectiveness

Rubella vaccine is a live attenuated virus vaccine (RA 27/3) prepared in human diploid cells. It is available as a monovalent (rubella only) vaccine as well as in combinations: measles and rubella, mumps and rubella, and measles, mumps, and rubella (MMR). In most circumstances, MMR is preferred.

A single dose of live attenuated rubella vaccine provides long-term (probably lifetime) immunity to more than 95% of recipients. Protection is effective against both clinical disease and asymptomatic viremia.

Although some vaccine recipients shed small amounts of vaccine virus from the pharynx, more than 20 years of experience provides good evidence that transmission does not occur. Thus, no contraindication to immunizing the contacts of pregnant women exists.

Indications

Rubella vaccine is recommended for adults, particularly women, unless there is proof of immunity (documented rubella vaccination on or after their first birthday, or a positive serologic test) or the vaccine is specifically contraindicated. In particular, susceptible women of childbearing age who are not pregnant should receive rubella vaccine during routine visits for medical and gynecologic care or family planning; after premarital screening; before discharge from a hospital for any reason; and in postpartum and postabortion settings. Every step should be taken to vaccinate women whenever they are exposed to the health care setting. Evidence of rubella immunity should be required for all persons in colleges and other postsecondary institutions.

All health care workers, both men and women, should be immune. Consideration should be given to making rubella immunity a condition for their employment. Assurance of their immunity should be provided during their training as health care workers. Finally, because the risk of acquiring rubella while traveling outside the United States is greater than the risk within the United States, all women making international trips, particularly those of childbearing age, should be immune.

Serologic testing can determine immunity. However, routine serologic testing of all women of childbearing age before vaccination to determine immunity is expensive and has been ineffective because of low rates of follow-up immunization. Accordingly, rubella vaccination of women who are not pregnant and have no history of vaccination is recommended without serologic testing.

Administration and Adverse Reactions

A single dose (0.5 mL) of reconstituted vaccine (preferably MMR) should be administered subcutaneously.

Adverse reactions occur only in susceptible persons. Those already immune to rubella at the time of vaccination are not at risk for developing adverse reactions. In large-scale field trials, as many as 40% of susceptible adults who were vaccinated experienced joint pain, mostly in small peripheral joints, the knees, or both. Outright arthritis occurs less frequently. Arthralgias and transient arthritis occur more frequently and tend to be more severe in susceptible women than in children. When joint symptoms or other types of pain and paresthesias occur, they generally begin 1 to 3 weeks after immunization, persist for 1 day to 3 weeks, and rarely recur. Adults with joint problems seldom must limit their work activities. Persistent joint symptoms among susceptible persons who are vaccinated, primarily adult women, have been reported. Controversy about their frequency exists; however, in comparative studies, the frequency of chronic joint complaints is substantially greater after natural infection than after vaccination. In one small study, 5% of susceptible women vaccinated, compared with 30% infected with wild-type virus, reported joint symptoms that persisted for at least 18 months. Transient peripheral neuritis and complaints such as paresthesias and pain in the arms and legs rarely occur.

Precautions and Contraindications

Because of the theoretical risk to the fetus, women of childbearing age should receive rubella vaccine only if they say they are not pregnant. They should be counseled not to become pregnant for 3 months after vaccination. Reasonable precautions include asking women if they are pregnant and explaining the theoretical risks of the vaccine. If a pregnant woman is vaccinated or becomes pregnant within 3 months of vaccination, she should be counseled about the theoretical risks to the fetus.

Through 1988, the Centers for Disease Control and Prevention prospectively monitored 321 susceptible pregnant women who had received rubella vaccine within 3 months before or after conception and who had carried their pregnancies to term. None of the infants had malformations associated with congenital rubella syndrome. The risk for rubella vaccine-associated malformation appears to be negligible. Although a final decision must rest with the patient and her physician, rubella vaccination during pregnancy should not ordinarily be a reason to recommend termination of the pregnancy.

Allergic reactions have not been reported with rubella vaccine, but the vaccine does contain trace amounts of neomycin, to which some patients may be allergic. Persons with a history of anaphylactic reactions (hives, swelling of the mouth and throat, difficulty in breathing, hypotension, or shock) after receiving neomycin should not receive rubella vaccine. Persons with reactions to neomycin that are not anaphylactic are not at increased risk and can be vaccinated.

Rubella vaccine should be given at least 14 days before or several months (Table 1.6) after administration of immune globulin, whole blood, or other blood products containing antibody (for example, human anti-Rho [D] globulin). However, previous administration of such blood products should not delay postpartum vaccination. Susceptible women should be vaccinated immediately after delivery and, if possible, tested at least 3 months later to determine immunity.

Rubella vaccine should not be given to persons who are immunocompromised as a result of most immunodeficiency diseases, leukemia, lymphoma, or generalized malignancy, or to persons who are immunosuppressed because of therapy with corticosteroids, alkylating drugs, antimetabolites, or radiation. However, persons with leukemia who are in remission and have not received chemotherapy for at least 3 months and asymptomatic persons with HIV may be vaccinated with rubella vaccine or MMR without adverse effects.

Revaccination

Revaccination is not recommended because immunity after a single dose of vaccine is thought to be lifelong. However, MMR is the preferred vaccine if measles or mumps vaccines are to be given. The administration of rubella vaccine to a person with either naturally acquired or vaccine-induced immunity is not associated with an increased risk for adverse reactions.

Unresolved Issues

Because MMR has been given without untoward incident in asymptomatic persons with HIV and persons with leukemia in remission, it is recommended for susceptible persons with these conditions. The risks and benefits of this vaccine in other conditions associated with immunocompromise are unknown.

The administration of rubella vaccine, either alone or as MMR, to susceptible adults commonly causes transient joint symptoms (arthralgias or arthritis). The role of this vaccine in causing chronic arthritis is controversial. Although women of childbearing potential and those in contact with such women should be immune to rubella, the benefits and risks of immunizing other susceptible adults with rubella vaccine are not entirely clear. However, MMR is recommended for those susceptible to rubella and for those in whom either measles or mumps vaccine is indicated for several reasons: because 1) most adults will have contact with pregnant women at some time; 2) the resurgence of rubella and congenital rubella in the 1980s and 1990s showed that rubella epidemics still occur; and 3) infection with wild-type virus is associated with a greater incidence of joint symptoms than is the vaccine.

Smallpox

In May 1980, the World Health Organization declared the world free of smallpox. In January 1982, smallpox was eliminated from the list of diseases subject to that organization's regulations. A smallpox vaccination certificate is no longer required by any country as a condition of entry for international travelers. In May 1983, distribution of smallpox vaccine for civilian use in the United States was discontinued.

Vaccine, Indications, Adverse Reactions, Precautions, and Contraindications

Smallpox vaccine is a live vaccinia virus vaccine. Except for persons working with orthopox viruses or those involved in the production and testing of smallpox vaccine, no indications exist for use of smallpox vaccine. For advice on vaccine administration and contraindications, contact the Drug Service of the Centers for Disease Control and Prevention in Atlanta, Georgia 30333 or call them at 404-639-3670 during the day or at 404-639-2888 in the evening and on weekends. No evidence exists that smallpox vaccination is valuable in treating recurrent herpes simplex virus infections, warts, or any other disease. Smallpox vaccine should never be used therapeutically.

In research studies, recombinant vaccinia virus is used as a vaccine to deliver other immunogens. Health care workers involved in these studies receive smallpox vaccine. In addition, the U.S. Armed Forces continue to administer smallpox vaccine to selected military personnel. Thus, a physician in civilian practice could encounter a patient with a complication of smallpox vaccination. Staff at the Centers for Disease Control and Prevention can assist in the diagnosis and management of such patients. Vaccinia immune globulin is available for use when indicated.

Unresolved Issues

The risks of complications from smallpox vaccination increase in persons who are immunocompromised, including those infected with HIV. Knowledge of the risks of inadvertent vaccination or secondary contact spread of vaccinia virus to these persons requires continuing evaluation and periodic reassessment of the current smallpox vaccination policy for military personnel.

Tetanus and Diphtheria

Tetanus

The incidence of tetanus in the United States has decreased dramatically so that only 45 to 65 cases have been reported annually in recent years. Almost all cases occur in persons who never completed a primary immunization series, did not receive appropriate treatment for a tetanus-prone wound, or both. Adults 60 years or older account for 60% of all tetanus cases. The overall case-fatality rate is approximately 31%, but it increases to 42% in persons 50 years or older. Among the patients who contract tetanus, despite having completed a primary immunization series (10% of the total), the disease is milder than in those who are less well immunized.

For persons who complete a primary series of three doses, booster doses of tetanus or tetanus-diphtheria (Td) toxoid reliably increase antibody levels even after intervals of 35 years or longer. In the United States, serologic studies indicate that at least 40% of persons 60 years or older do not have protective serum levels of antitoxin. In addition, approximately 11% of adults ages 18 to 39 years lack what are considered to be protective levels of circulating antitoxin. These data indicate poor compliance with the current recommendations for universal primary vaccination and for booster doses of tetanus toxoid every 10 years. Despite this evidence of adult susceptibility, cases of tetanus are rare among adults who have, at any previous time, received a complete primary series. Thus, although seroprevalence studies are cited in support of the current policy of routine tetanus boosters every 10 years for all adults, the clinical epidemiologic evidence indicates that routine booster doses are of marginal value. Rather, physicians should ensure that all patients receive a primary immunization series and promote Td boosters for patients with tetanus-prone wounds. Pregnant women who are not fully immunized are also prime candidates for immunization to protect themselves and their newborns.

Diphtheria

Widespread use of diphtheria toxoid has eliminated respiratory diphtheria from the United States. Nonetheless, a few cases (five or fewer) are reported each year, most of which occur in persons who are unimmunized or inadequately immunized. The case-fatality rate for diphtheria is 5% to 10%, although no deaths have been reported in the past decade. Diphtheria is predominately a disease of adults; of the 40 cases of respiratory diphtheria reported during the 13-year period from 1980 to 1992, most occurred in persons 20 years or older.

Because of effective pediatric immunization programs, most children have adequate protection against diphtheria. After a person completes a primary series, a booster dose elicits a brisk antibody response even many years later. However, serologic studies indicate that 62% of adults 18 to 39 years old and 41% to 84% of those 60 years or older lack protective levels of circulating antitoxin. The serologic evidence of susceptibility among adults reflects diminished natural exposure to infection and poor compliance with the recommendation that adults receive booster injections of diphtheria toxoid every 10 years throughout their lives. Despite this evidence of adult susceptibility, cases of diphtheria are rare among adults who have ever received a complete primary series, suggesting that routine booster immunizations have a marginal effect. Among the few patients (average, one per year since 1980) who contracted diphtheria, despite a history suggesting previous immunization, the disease was milder, and no deaths occurred.

Tetanus and Diphtheria Toxoids, Clinical Effectiveness, Indications, Administration, and Reimmunization

Tetanus and diphtheria are completely preventable, and everyone should be actively immunized against both diseases. The combined Td toxoid, adsorbed, (5 Lf units tetanus toxoid and 2 Lf units of diphtheria toxoid per 0.5-mL dose) is the preferred preparation for active tetanus and diphtheria immunization of adults. A primary series consists of two doses (0.5 mL each) given intramuscularly at least 4 weeks apart, followed by a third dose (0.5 mL) given 6 to 12 months later. All adults who have not received at least three doses of tetanus and diphtheria toxoids should complete a primary series with combined Td toxoid. Doses do not need to be repeated if the schedule for the primary series has been delayed. A booster dose given as long as 25 to 30 years after primary vaccination produces a rapid and significant increase in levels of circulating antitoxins against both tetanus and diphtheria.

The traditional recommendation for Td boosters is that all adults receive a Td booster every 10 years throughout their lives. While endorsing this policy, the Task Force on Adult Immunization recommends as an equivalent alternative strategy that special emphasis be given to the completion of a primary immunization series with tetanus and diphtheria toxoids followed by a single booster at age 50 years for persons who have completed the full pediatric series, including the teenage and young adult booster. The Task Force believes that this specific age recommendation may result in better compliance by physicians and patients. Neither the dicennial booster policy nor the single mid-life Td booster policy affect the need to give a

Td booster as part of wound management. The Task Force on Adult Immunization strongly recommends age 50 years as an ideal time to review immunization status and other preventive measures. In addition to a Td booster, an assessment should be made regarding risk factors that would indicate a need for pneumococcal vaccine, annual influenza immunization, or both.

Tetanus Immune Globulin and Diphtheria Antitoxin

Human tetanus immune globulin is highly protective when given for passive immunization against tetanus. The recommended dose is 250 U administered intramuscularly. After injection, protective levels of antitoxin are present in all patients for 28 days and in 84% of patients after 8 weeks. When given with tetanus toxoid, separate syringes and separate injection sites should be used. Diphtheria antitoxin of equine origin is available for the early treatment of respiratory diphtheria and can be obtained from the manufacturer (*see* Appendix 2). It probably has no value for cutaneous diphtheria. The administration and dose vary by situation.

Special Indication: Wound Management

The indications for active and passive immunization against tetanus in the management of wounds are summarized in Table 5.1.

Cases of tetanus have occurred rarely in persons with a documented primary series of tetanus toxoid. A completed primary series provides protection for 10 or more years in almost all recipients. For minor wounds that are clean, a booster dose of tetanus toxoid is needed only if 10 years have passed since completion of the primary series or the last booster dose. For more severe, contaminated wounds, a booster dose is indicated if more than 5 years have passed.

Every effort should be made to determine whether the patient has completed a primary series of immunization with tetanus toxoid and, if the series is incomplete, how many doses were given. Passive immunization with tetanus immune globulin may be required in addition to tetanus toxoid for persons whose immunization status is incomplete, unknown, or uncertain. Adsorbed, not fluid, tetanus toxoid should be used if tetanus immune globulin is given.

In managing wounds, combined Td toxoid should be used to increase the level of immunity to diphtheria as well as to tetanus. A primary series of combined tetanus and diphtheria toxoid should be completed in anyone who has never been immunized or whose immunization status is uncertain.

Adverse Reactions

Local erythema and induration, with or without tenderness, can occur after the administration of combined Td toxoid. Fever and other systemic reactions are uncommon unless the person has been hyperimmunized. In many such cases, a characteristic Arthur-type hypersensitivity reaction appears 2 to 8 hours after injection. Although it causes local discomfort, it is rarely serious. These reactions usually occur in persons who have high serum anti-toxin levels. Anyone who has ever had such a reaction should be instructed not to receive booster doses of combined Td more often than once every 10 years. However, whenever a tetanus booster is indicated, combined Td toxoid should be used rather than tetanus toxoid alone; the addition of diphtheria toxoid does not increase the rate of adverse reactions.

Severe systemic reactions such as anaphylaxis, generalized urticaria, angioedema, or neurologic complications have been reported rarely. A causal relationship between neurologic reactions and the administration of tetanus and diphtheria toxoids has not been established.

Precautions and Contraindications

The only contraindication to administering combined Td toxoid is a history of a severe hypersensitivity or neurologic reaction after a previous dose. Local side effects alone do not preclude booster injections at 10-year intervals. If an anaphylactic reaction to a previous dose is suspected, intradermal skin testing with appropriately diluted toxoid should be carefully done before tetanus immunization is discontinued. Nonspecific skin test reactivity to tetanus and diphtheria toxoids develops in most persons. Thus, a negative skin test result is unusual. However, a positive skin test result without a history of clinical symptoms of severe allergic reaction is not a sufficient reason to omit or defer scheduled doses of combined Td toxoid.

Pregnant women should be kept current regarding Td immunizations so they confer protection against tetanus and diphtheria on their infants by placental transfer of maternal antibodies.

Unresolved Issues

In the United States, older adults who have not received a primary series of immunizations are the primary population at risk for tetanus and diphtheria. Physicians must take advantage of every medical encounter with adults to review and, when appropriate, immunize with combined Td to ensure adequate protection against these diseases.

Tuberculosis

From 1963 to 1985, the incidence of tuberculosis in the United States declined an average of 6% each year. The decline stopped in 1985, and since then increasing rates of new cases of active tuberculosis have been recorded each year. In 1990, the increase was 9.4%, the largest annual increase in nearly 40 years. The greatest increase occurred among younger adults 25 to 44 years old. Both newly acquired and reactivation tuberculosis in patients with HIV infection accounted for most of this increase. For this reason, all persons with newly diagnosed tuberculosis should be tested for HIV infection and, conversely, persons with HIV infection should be given tuberculin skin tests. Although some HIV-infected patients may be anergic, a positive skin test result is meaningful. Other groups at high risk for infection with tuberculosis include immigrants and refugees who have recently arrived from areas with a high prevalence of disease, homeless persons, and members of minority groups.

Recently, drug-resistant tubercle bacilli have become an important concern. During the first quarter of 1991, 13% of new cases of tuberculosis were caused by strains resistant to at least one antituberculosis drug. Some strains were resistant to multiple drugs (MDR-TB). Outbreaks of MDR-TB have occurred in several hospitals and a state prison system.

Bacille Calmette-Guérin Vaccine, Clinical Effectiveness, and Indications

Live Bacille Calmette-Guérin (BCG) vaccines are used throughout the world to prevent tuberculosis in children. However, field trials in adults have yielded disparate and conflicting results.

Bacille Calmette-Guérin vaccination is not recommended for health care workers or for other adults at high risk for acquiring tuberculosis. One of its drawbacks is that it reduces the tuberculin skin test's ability to detect recent acquisition of *Mycobacterium tuberculosis* infection. Health care workers should be adequately protected by periodic tuberculin skin testing and isoniazid preventive therapy for all skin-test- positive persons at risk for acquiring the disease. In health care settings where MDR-TB is prevalent, BCG vaccine may be considered on a case-by-case basis for administration to immunocompetent, tuberculin-negative health care personnel who will be at continuing risk for exposure.

In the United States, BCG vaccination might be considered for infants and children who are skin-test negative and who 1) cannot receive isoniazid preventive therapy but have close contact with patients with active tuberculosis that is untreated, ineffectively treated, or resistant to isoniazid and rifampin; or 2) belong to groups in which an excessive rate of new infections (more than 1% per year) can be shown and the usual surveillance and treatment programs have failed or are not feasible.

Administration, Adverse Reactions, Precautions, and Contraindications

In the United States, BCG vaccine is licensed only for intradermal administration. It should be given only by the route specified in the package insert.

Bacille Calmette-Guérin vaccination has been associated with prolonged purulent discharge and ulceration at the vaccination site, regional adenitis, and osteitis. Ulceration and adenitis can occur in more than 20% of vaccinated persons. In those with active tuberculosis, the response to BCG vaccine is accelerated, with induration and pustule formation appearing 1 week rather than 2 to 3 weeks after vaccination. Disseminated BCG infections and death are rare (1 to 10 per 10 million vaccinated persons) and almost always occur in persons who are immunocompromised.

Although no harmful effects of BCG vaccine on the fetus have been observed, it is prudent not to vaccinate women during pregnancy. Because BCG vaccine is a live bacterial vaccine, it should not be given to persons who are immunocompromised because of congenital or acquired immunodeficiency diseases (including HIV infection), leukemia, lymphoma, or generalized malignancy, or to persons who are immunosuppressed by therapy with corticosteroids, alkylating agents, antimetabolites, or radiation.

Interpretation of Tuberculin Skin Tests after BCG Vaccination

It is impossible to determine whether a positive tuberculin skin test is caused by mycobacterial infection or by BCG vaccination itself in persons who received BCG vaccine. The likelihood that a positive skin test result indicates exposure to *M. tuberculosis* increases 1) as the size of the reaction increases; 2) when there has been contact with a person with tuberculosis who has infected others; 3) when there is a family history of tuberculosis; 4) if the person's country of origin has a high prevalence of tuberculosis; and 5) when the length of time between vaccination and tuberculin skin testing increases. Thus, for example, a positive skin test (induration measuring 10 mm or more) in a BCG-vaccinated person is more likely to be caused by infection with *M. tuberculosis* if the person was knowingly exposed to someone with infectious tuberculosis or is in a group at high risk for tuberculosis. However, in a person without such exposure who is not in a high-risk group, a positive skin test may not indicate recent infection with *M. tuberculosis*. Nonetheless, tuberculosis should be considered in the differential diagnosis of any tuberculosis-like illness, regardless of previous BCG vaccination.

Unresolved Issues

The efficacy of BCG in preventing pulmonary tuberculosis in adults remains unresolved. Under debate is whether health care workers (some of whom may be HIV infected) in areas of high endemicity for MDR-TB should be vaccinated with BCG. The resurgence of tuberculosis has rekindled interest in developing new and better immunogens.

Typhoid

Typhoid fever is a systemic febrile illness cause by *Salmonella typhi*. In contrast to other *Salmonella* species, humans are the only reservoir for *S. typhi*. Infection is almost always a consequence of ingesting contaminated food, water, or milk. Most of the approximately 500 cases of typhoid reported in the United States each year are acquired abroad.

Vaccine, Clinical Effectiveness, and Indications

Three inactivated parenteral typhoid vaccines and one oral live attenuated vaccine are manufactured. The three parenteral vaccines are 1) a heat-phenol-treated vaccine (the older commercially available vaccine); 2) an acetone-treated vaccine (available only for the Armed Forces); and 3) the Vi capsular polysaccharide vaccine (ViCPS), which is composed of purified Vi ("virulence") antigen that is the capsular polysaccharide elaborated by bloodstream isolates of *Salmonella typhi*. Antibodies to Vi are associated with typhoid fever protection. Compared with the older parenteral typhoid vaccines, ViCPS results in an equivalent immune response and protective efficacy and has fewer side effects.

A single 25-μg injection of the new ViCPS produced seroconversion in 83% to 98% of healthy U.S. adult volunteers. In Nepal, one dose provided 74% protection against blood culture-confirmed typhoid fever.

The oral vaccine is a live attenuated Ty21a strain of *S. typhi*. In clinical trials, three doses of oral vaccine were 67% effective in reducing laboratory-confirmed infection. In another trial, four doses were more effective than three doses in preventing disease. The oral vaccine has few side effects and confers protection equivalent to the parenteral vaccines.

Vaccines against paratyphoid A and B are no longer included in typhoid vaccines because of lack of efficacy and additive side effects of the paratyphoid components.

Typhoid vaccination is not required for international travel. The decision to immunize a traveler should be based on consideration of the itinerary, the duration and style of travel, and the willingness of the traveler to accept risk. For travelers on short trips who are careful about what they eat and drink, immunization is generally not necessary.

Travelers who expect prolonged exposure to potentially contaminated food and drink are candidates for vaccination. High-risk areas are developing countries (especially in Latin America, Asia, and Africa). Vaccination, however, is not a substitute for observing food and drink precautions because a high inoculum of *S. typhi* can overwhelm vaccine-induced immunity. In addition, potential contamination of food and drink by other enteric pathogens are not prevented by typhoid vaccine.

In the United States, vaccine is recommended only for continued household contact with *S. typhi* carriers and for microbiology laboratory workers frequently exposed to *S. typhi*. It is not recommended after flooding or other natural disasters.

Administration, Adverse Reactions, Precautions, and Contraindications

The oral vaccine primary dosage schedule is one enteric-coated capsule taken on alternate days for a total of four capsules. The capsule is given with a cool liquid 1 hour before a meal. Capsules are kept refrigerated before use. Adverse reactions to the oral vaccine are unusual. Viable organisms are not shed in the stool. The live vaccine should not be given to immunocompromised patients, including those infected with the human immunodeficiency virus; rather, the killed vaccine is preferred for those persons.

The oral vaccine should not be given during an acute episode of diarrhea or when the patient is receiving antimicrobial agents. Mefloquine may decrease the immune response if given with the oral vaccine; it should be taken at least 24 hours before ingesting an oral vaccine capsule. Administration of immunoglobulin will not decrease the immunogenicity of the live Ty21a vaccine.

The primary series for the new Vi capsular polysaccharide parenteral vaccine is a single intramuscular dose of 25 μg (0.5 mL) and has minimal side effects. Therefore, it is preferred to the heat-phenol-treated parenteral vaccine, which requires two doses (0.5 mL each) administered subcutaneously 4 or more weeks apart and commonly causes systemic illness and discomfort at the site of injection. These symptoms are attributed to endotoxin in the heat-phenol vaccine. A severe local or systemic reaction to previous typhoid immunization is a contraindication to further administration of heat-phenol typhoid vaccine but should not preclude use of the oral attenuated vaccine or ViCPS.

Revaccination

Revaccination with four doses of the oral vaccine every 5 years is recommended for repeated exposure to *S. typhi*. The optimal booster schedule, however, has not been determined, and the interval may change.

A single booster dose of 0.5 mL (25 mg) of the parenteral ViCPS vaccine is recommended every 2 years after the primary dose when continued or renewed exposure is expected. For the heat-phenol-treated parenteral vaccine, a booster dose (0.5 mL) administered subcutaneously is indicated every 3 years only if continued or repeated exposure to *S. typhi* is expected. Intradermal injection (0.1 mL) may be preferred to the larger subcutaneous dose because it causes fewer incidents of fever and local irritation. However, the acetone-killed vaccine, available only to U.S. military personnel, should not be given intradermally.

No experience has been reported on the effect of administering ViCPS or Ty21a as a booster to persons previously vaccinated with the heat-phenol-treated parenteral vaccine, but it is a reasonable alternative to the heat-phenol-treated vaccine.

Unresolved Issues

The ViCPS vaccine is at least comparable to the previously available vaccines and has the advantage of single-dose administration and negligible side effects. If it is competitively priced, it will probably become the standard typhoid vaccine.

Varicella Zoster

Most adults (85% to 95%) with negative or unknown histories of varicella (chicken pox) are probably immune. Primary varicella is usually more severe in adults than it is in healthy children; in immunocompromised, susceptible adults, an even greater risk of serious complications or death exists.

Varicella Zoster Immune Globulin, Clinical Effectiveness, Indications, Administration, and Adverse Reactions

If, on the basis of a carefully obtained history, an immunocompromised patient is believed to be susceptible to varicella and has had substantial exposure, varicella zoster immune globulin (VZIG) should be given. Substantial exposures include household contacts; close indoor contact lasting more than 1 hour; sharing the same two- to four-bed hospital room with an infected person; or prolonged, direct, face-to-face contact with an infected person, such as occurs with nurses or physicians.

Pregnant women in whom varicella (but not herpes zoster) develops may have an increased risk for severe pneumonia or premature labor. Administration of VZIG may prevent or modify serious maternal illness, although it will not prevent intrauterine infection. Infants born to mothers in whom varicella develops within 5 days before or 48 hours after delivery should receive VZIG to reduce the likelihood of acquiring serious or fatal neonatal varicella. Pregnant, varicella-susceptible women exposed to varicella may also be given VZIG to modify the severity of illness.

All decisions to administer VZIG to healthy adults should be evaluated individually. Serologic testing, if available, may help determine susceptibility. Varicella zoster immune globulin is available through selected American Red Cross distribution centers and is supplied in 125-U vials. Supplies are limited, and indiscriminate use in healthy adults could quickly exhaust supplies and prevent the more urgent prophylaxis of immunocompromised persons. Also, an adult dose of five vials is expensive, approximately $500. An acceptable alternative is not to test for immunity or give VZIG prophylaxis, but instead to treat varicella, if it occurs, with oral or intravenous acyclovir. Because of concerns about adverse effects on the fetus, acyclovir is recommended in pregnant women only as a life-saving measure. Health care personnel known to be susceptible should be evaluated in the same way as other adults and should be removed from duty during the incubation period, which is 8 to 21 days after exposure.

No data provide a basis for determining the appropriate dose of VZIG for immunocompromised adults. Whereas 125 U/10 kg (up to a maximum of 625 U) is considered adequate for healthy adults, higher doses may be necessary for those who are immunocompromised. The VZIG should be administered intramuscularly. Although the duration of protection is unknown, it should last for 1 half-life of the immune globulin, that is, approximately 3 weeks. Serious adverse effects from immune globulins administered as recommended have been rare.

Varicella Vaccine

A live attenuated varicella vaccine (Oka strain) has been used widely in Japan and selectively in Europe for more than a decade. Licensure in the United States is probable in the near future, with the primary target group being healthy children, in whom levels of complete protection exceed 85%. The vaccine has few adverse reactions, the most common being local reaction, an attenuated rash, and mild fever. It has been well tolerated and protective in immunocompromised patients, who bear the greatest risk of acquiring severe varicella. The incidence of zoster is not increased in healthy immunized children and is lower in vaccinated children with leukemia than in persons with leukemia who have had natural varicella.

Among adults, the vaccine is less immunogenic as measured by humoral antibodies and cell-mediated immunity; therefore a two-dose immunization schedule is required. In several small studies, vaccination of healthy adults prevented clinical illness after exposure to varicella or modified the severity of illness in all cases. When licensed, the vaccine will be targeted for certain seronegative adults, particularly those working in health care, teachers, and others with frequent exposure to children. Immunization of susceptible nonpregnant women of childbearing age would protect against future perinatal exposure of their infants and against the severe illness that often characterizes varicella during pregnancy. Although postexposure vaccination within 3 days of contact with the index case has prevented development of varicella in 90% to 100% of healthy children, extrapolation to adults is not warranted because of the lower immunogenicity of the vaccine in adults. Studies of the vaccine's effect in ameliorating the incidence and severity of zoster are underway in adults who had varicella infection as children.

Yellow Fever

Yellow fever is a severe, hemorrhagic viral illness transmitted by *Aedes* species mosquitoes. Although conditions necessary for transmission are present throughout the tropics and subtropics, cases are reported only from equatorial Africa and from South America and Panama, with some extensions into Trinidad. Yellow fever has not been documented among U.S. travelers in more than 50 years, although European travelers have contracted yellow fever during visits to Africa in the 1980s.

Vaccine, Clinical Effectiveness, and Indications

Yellow fever vaccine is a live attenuated virus vaccine prepared from the 17D strain of virus grown in chick embryo. The vaccine virus is highly temperature sensitive and must be kept frozen during transportation and storage. Once reconstituted, it must be used within 60 minutes. In the United States, only health facilities that agree to meet stringent conditions regarding transportation, handling, storage, and administration of the vaccine have been designated Yellow Fever Vaccination Centers. Yellow fever vaccine is highly immunogenic and is believed to be very effective in preventing the disease.

Vaccination is recommended for persons traveling or living in areas where yellow fever infection occurs. A valid International Certificate of Vaccination is a requirement for entry into certain countries where yellow fever occurs, particularly if the traveler is arriving from an endemic area. Information regarding infected areas is published annually in *Health Information for International Travel.* Countries reporting yellow fever are noted biweekly in *Summary of Health Information for International Travel.* Both publications are received by all state and many county and city health departments. Specific advice on yellow fever risks and immunization can be obtained from the Centers for Disease Control and Prevention, Fort Collins, Colorado (303-221-6400).

Vaccination is also recommended for laboratory personnel who might be exposed to wild-type and vaccine strains of yellow fever virus.

Administration and Adverse Reactions

A single dose (0.5 mL) of reconstituted yellow fever vaccine given subcutaneously is adequate for primary immunization. Travelers who are vaccinated should also receive a signed and stamped International Certificate of Vaccination. The certificate is valid for 10 years, beginning 10 days after primary immunization and immediately after revaccination.

Reactions to yellow fever vaccine are generally mild. From 2% to 5% of vaccinated persons develop mild headache, myalgia, low-grade fever, and other minor symptoms 5 to 10 days after vaccination. Fewer than 0.2% must limit their regular activities. Immediate hypersensitivity reactions (rash, urticaria, and asthma, for example) are very rare and occur primarily in persons who are allergic to eggs. Vaccine-related encephalitis is rare and occurs primarily in children younger than 4 months old. More than 200 million doses of vaccine have been distributed worldwide, and only 18 cases of postvaccinal encephalitis have been reported since 1945.

Precautions and Contraindications

Yellow fever vaccine generally should not be given to persons who are immunocompromised as a result of immunodeficiency diseases (including HIV infection), leukemia, lymphoma, or generalized malignancy or who are immunosuppressed as a result of therapy with corticosteroids, alkylating drugs, antimetabolites, or radiation.

Although specific information is not available regarding adverse effects of yellow fever vaccine on the developing fetus, it is prudent to avoid vaccinating pregnant women and to advise postponing travel to areas where yellow fever occurs until after delivery. However, for pregnant women who must travel to areas where the risk for yellow fever is high, immunization is recommended because the risk for infection is believed to outweigh the small theoretical risk from vaccination.

Because yellow fever vaccine is produced in chick embryos, persons with a history of anaphylactic hypersensitivity to eggs should not be vaccinated. Infants younger than 6 months are more susceptible to serious adverse reactions (encephalitis) than are older children and thus should not be immunized. The risk for serious complications in infants appears to be age related. Whenever possible, vaccination should be delayed until at least 12 months of age.

Studies suggest that lower than normal antibody responses to both vaccines develop in persons given yellow fever and injectable whole-cell cholera vaccines simultaneously or 1 to 3 weeks apart. Unless there are time constraints, the two vaccines should be administered separately at least 3 weeks apart. If the vaccines cannot be administered in that time frame, they should be given simultaneously. Yellow fever vaccine can be given simultaneously with as much as 5 mL of immune globulin without losing its effectiveness. Chloroquine inhibits the replication of yellow fever virus *in vitro* but does not adversely affect the antibody response to the vaccine in persons who are taking chloroquine as antimalarial prophylaxis.

Revaccination

In persons with continued exposure to yellow fever, a booster dose (0.5 mL given subcutaneously) is indicated at 10-year intervals.

9.

Future Trends in Vaccine Development and Delivery

New techniques in molecular biology have brought rapid progress in the development of vaccines. Several recently released or soon-to-be-licensed vaccines reflect this new technology, and many diseases have, for the first time, become targets for vaccine prevention. These technical developments stand in striking contrast to the inadequacies of our efforts to deliver already-existing vaccines indicated for adults.

New Technologies for Producing Vaccines

Until recently, methods to develop live attenuated virus vaccines were limited to serial passage in cell culture (oral polio vaccine), variant viruses from other species (vaccinia virus for smallpox vaccine), and temperature-selective mutants and genetic reassortments (influenza vaccine). Live attenuated virus vaccines generally provide long-lasting protection, but in certain instances they may cause adverse reactions or revert, rarely, to more pathogenic forms. Newer techniques have made it possible to identify regions of viral genomes that, if altered, lead to attenuation. By deleting elements of the genome essential to viral virulence, reversion can be prevented. This approach is being used to develop a safer live attenuated oral type 3 polio vaccine. Another method that could have broad applications is genetic alteration of a live virus, such as vaccinia virus, so it functions as a carrier for genes that code for several antigenic proteins (for example, hepatitis B surface antigen). Enthusiasm for using vaccinia virus to immunize against several diseases simultaneously is tempered by concern about its potential for causing adverse reactions, especially in persons who are immunocompromised. Nonreplicating avian pox viruses offer the possibility of a safer vaccine.

Killed vaccines were made initially from whole-cell pathogens (for example, typhoid, and cholera) or their toxoids. More recently, purified surface components have been used, either alone (for example, pneumococcal vaccine) or conjugated to carrier proteins such as diphtheria toxoid (for example, *Haemophilus influenzae* type b vaccine). Recombinant DNA techniques have made it possible to isolate genes encoding for protective antigens and to express them in other host cells. This approach has been used to produce a yeast-cell-derived recombinant hepatitis B vaccine. Special techniques have also permitted the identification and isolation of shorter genetic sequences that can be used, in turn, to synthesize large amounts of specific oligopeptides. Because of the complexity of most antigens, these synthetic peptide vaccines are often less immunogenic than their parent antigens. Efforts have been made to increase the immunogenicity of these synthetic antigens by incorporating them into adjuvants, by coupling to carrier proteins, or by creating antigen presentation systems such as immunostimulating complexes and virus-like protein particles. Anti-idiotype antibodies used with some antigens as vaccines someday may also be successful. Theoretically, the anti-idiotype antibodies produced should carry antigenic specificity identical to that of the primary antigen.

New Vaccines

In 1986, the National Institute of Allergy and Infectious Diseases targeted seven vaccines for priority development. Of these, two have since been licensed (recombinant hepatitis B and *H. influenzae* type b conjugate vaccines), and another (varicella vaccine) should be licensed soon. Some research progress has been made with live attenuated (cold adapted *[ca]*) influenza vaccine and respiratory syncytial virus vaccine. Important obstacles, principally antigenic diversity among strains, have thwarted progress to develop an effective gonococcal vaccine. Some recent developments with several of these and other vaccines that are in Phase 1, 2, or 3 trials but have not yet been licensed are worth reviewing. Vaccines that are being studied in animal models and have not yet reached Phase 1 trials in humans will be excluded from further discussion here.

Respiratory Virus Infections

For more than two decades, the inability of inactivated influenza vaccines to confer prolonged, high-level protection has stimulated efforts to develop attenuated live virus vaccines. Current research includes use of *ca* live mutants administered with nose drops. Clinical trials have shown that they may be effective in preventing acute infections but are not of decidedly superior efficacy when compared with conventional inactivated vaccines. Furthermore, the long-term safety of yearly immunization of high-risk persons with live virus preparations is problematic. Many other approaches to influenza vaccine development are being tried. Influenza virus genes can be introduced into vaccine vectors to carry foreign genes for influenza and other respiratory pathogens. Alternative delivery strategies, such as microencapsulation and addition of conventional adjuvants, may improve the immune response. Stimulation of cytotoxic T lymphocytes with antigen formulations that permit class I responses may permit cellular immune responses. Using highly conserved amino-acid sequences in the hemagglutinin or in the nucleoprotein as immunogen may induce cross-reactive protection. The control of influenza virus infection, however, will always be a challenge because the virus changes its critical surface antigens almost every year (drift) or makes major periodic changes after long intervals (shift).

Parainfluenza virus (PI) type 3 *ca* mutants are being investigated, as is a bovine strain (PI3) of virus that is antigenically related to human strains. For respiratory syncytial virus, a purified F (fusion) surface glycoprotein vaccine was tested in children without adverse effects. Studies to rule out their ability to potentiate naturally occurring disease are being done.

Researchers are trying to develop vaccines that can be given at age 6 months, even in the presence of maternal antibody.

Respiratory Bacterial Infections

The vaccine against *H. influenzae* type b (Hib) was the first to incorporate the concept of covalently linking a protein carrier to the bacterium's capsular polysaccharide to enhance its immunogenicity. Four vaccines of this type have been licensed. They differ in the size of the polysaccharide, type of protein carrier, and chemical form of covalent linkage. Other Hib-conjugated vaccines are being investigated.

Protective efficacy of conventional pneumococcal vaccines may not be adequate, especially in children younger than 2 years, and has led to a search for more effective vaccines. Protein-conjugated *Streptococcus pneumoniae* polysaccharide vaccine development is being pursued using the technology developed for the *H. influenzae* type b conjugated vaccines. The polysaccharides of pneumococcal strains 6B, 14, 19, and 23F have been conjugated to one of the following proteins: meningococcal group B outer membrane protein, tetanus toxoid, or the diphtheria toxin cross-reactive protein CRM 197. Three different glycoconjugate pneumococcal vaccines are currently being tested in human trials.

Group B streptococcal infections are a common cause of neonatal illness and death. Neonatal immunity results from transfer of maternal antibody across the placenta; the infant is susceptible to disease when this immunity is absent. Glycoconjugate vaccines are being tested that contain type Ia, Ib, II, and III polysaccharide or oligosaccharide derivatives linked to a carrier protein. They are intended for use in pregnant mothers or in early infancy.

The licensed *Neisseria meningitidis* vaccine does not provide long-lasting immunity, and booster responses are poor. Glycoconjugate vaccines are being studied. Covalently linking meningococcal group A and C polysaccharides to a protein carrier would elicit a T-helper cell-dependent immune response that should enhance the overall immunogenicity of the two polysaccharides and provide immunologic memory. The group B polysaccharide presents a different problem. The antibody to group B polysaccharide does not appear to be protective. Alternative group B protein antigens, such as outer membrane protein and others, are being tested.

Less toxic acellular pertussis vaccines were recently licensed for booster immunization. Ongoing studies continue to examine the optimal vaccine composition for the four purified or recombinant pertussis antigens-pertussin toxin, filamentous hemagglutinin, pertactin outer membrane protein, and agglutinogens 2 and 3. The ability to synthesize nontoxic pertussin toxin molecules by making an enzymatically inactive S1 subunit has eliminated the ability to induce lymphocytosis, sensitize to histamine, activate islets, and potentiate anaphylaxis.

Hepatitis A

The propagation of hepatitis A in cell culture in 1979 paved the way for development of both live attenuated and killed hepatitis A vaccines. Two formalin-inactivated whole-virus vaccines are nearing licensure in the United States. In pediatric populations, protective rates greater than 95% have been reported after three doses in a Thai trial and after a single dose in a smaller U.S. trial. The vaccines appear to be very well tolerated, and although the duration of protection is unknown, antibody levels persist for at least several years. It is anticipated that when hepatitis A vaccine(s) becomes available, universal immunization of children may be recommended. Adults who may be targeted for hepatitis A vaccine could include international travelers, staff of day-care or custodial-care facilities, military personnel, food handlers, populations with high endemicity of infection (for example, American Indians and Alaskan natives), and persons whose sexual practices (male homosexuality or multiple sexual partners, for instance) place them at increased risk. Whether hepatitis A immunization will be valuable in the postexposure care of persons in contact with hepatitis A patients is not known. However, in all other settings, hepatitis A vaccines should eventually replace immunoglobulin to prevent hepatitis A.

Herpes Virus Infections

The ability of herpes viruses to produce latent infection poses a formidable challenge to vaccine development. The development of neutralizing antibody is not as effective in preventing disease as it is with other common viral infections, such as measles and polio, that have no latent phase. Because latent infection in ganglia provides a continuing reservoir of virus that can be reactivated, even in the presence of neutralizing antibody, preventing the initial infection from becoming latent is critical.

Substantial progress has been made in developing a varicella zoster vaccine. A live attenuated varicella vaccine (Oka vaccine) was developed in Japan and is licensed there and in several other countries. The vaccine should be licensed soon in the United States for use in healthy children and adults. Patients with leukemia can also be immunized with the vaccine under controlled circumstances. When the vaccine is given to adults older than 55 years, it increases anti-VZV antibody levels and VZV-specific T cells to levels seen in persons 20 years younger. The duration of immunity is uncertain. Zoster can develop in vaccinated persons, especially in children with leukemia, but the incidence appears to be less than that seen after wild-type infection.

Vaccination against primary cytomegalovirus infections to prevent fetal infection in susceptible pregnant women is needed, as is immunization of seronegative patients before they have organ transplants and immunosuppressive therapy. Clinical studies of the live attenuated Towne strain of cytomegalovirus have shown it to be antigenic and partially protective in renal transplant recipients. The vaccine virus is not excreted after inoculation, and latent infection is not established. Future vaccine development should incorporate the multiple strains of cytomegalovirus that have been described.

Several approaches are being investigated for infections caused by herpes simplex viruses (HSV) types 1 and 2. Prevention of HSV-2 rather than HSV-1 infection is the most urgent goal because recurrent genital herpes with HSV-2 can be debilitating and because consequences of neonatal infection can be devastating. Prevention and amelioration of the primary infection and modification of recurrent infections are being examined. Live attenuated virus and infected cell extracts as vaccines have been tested. A recombinant yeast-derived gD viral glycoprotein subunit vaccine shows promise. Most intriguing is a live attenuated HSV-1 vaccine that has a number of gene insertions and deletions. Sequences of HSV-2 glycoproteins (gD, gG, gE, and gI) were inserted into the HSV-1 genome. This genetic modification produced a virus that is unable to cause latency or central nervous system disease. The thymidine kinase gene remains in the genome and thus acyclovir sensitivity is retained. Phase 1 clinical trials show that the vaccine is immunogenic and does not cause adverse clinical effects.

Epstein-Barr virus is associated not only with the infectious mononucleosis syndrome but also with nasopharyngeal carcinoma, Burkitt lymphoma, and rarely chronic infection. High antibody-dependent cellular cytotoxicity titers to the Epstein-Barr virus membrane complex that contains gp 350, the major viral surface glycoprotein, is associated with a better prognosis in patients with nasopharyngeal carcinoma. Use of a vaccinia vector vaccine that expresses gp 350 has been proposed to halt the progression of nasopharyngeal carcinoma.

Enteric Infections

Theoretically, oral immunization should be preferred to prevent infection with enteric pathogens because it might provide greater protective intestinal immunity by stimulating local secretory IgA antibody than vaccines given parenterally. However, some parenteral vaccines may also provide protection against enteric infections, probably because pathogen-specific serum IgG antibody is secreted into the intestinal lumen. Development of more stable, live attenuated oral vaccines and less reactogenic parenteral vaccines is being pursued.

Oral genetically engineered *S. typhi* vaccines are being produced with deletions in critical metabolic pathways. Parenteral vaccines comprising purified virulence (Vi) carbohydrate antigens alone or conjugated to tetanus toxoid or cholera toxin show promise. The purified Vi antigen alone was 72% to 80% effective in Nepal and South Africa, where the endemic infection rate is high. It was also nonreactogenic. The vaccine is licensed outside the United States.

Knowledge that natural infection with *Vibrio cholera* is followed by long-lasting immunity has encouraged the development of several types of oral cholera vaccine. The first type uses inactivated, whole *V. cholerae* combined with either a chemically and heat-treated toxin (procholeragenoid) or a purified B subunit of the toxin. Vaccine with the B subunit was 50% protective overall for three seasons but poorly protective in children. The second vaccine type uses live attenuated, genetically altered *V. cholerae* strains (deletion or auxotrophic mutants). The CVD 103 HgR vaccine is a derivative of the Inaba strain of *V. cholerae*. The vaccine induces vibriocidal and antitoxin antibodies in 95% of recipients. The protective efficacy against the parent Inaba strain is 90% effective, and 67% to 78% effective against the related El Tor and Ogawa strains. Diarrhea was a side effect in 2% of vaccinated persons. A third type of vaccine is made of genetically engineered hybrid strains that express *V. cholerae* genes carried in other enteric pathogens, such as *E. coli* K-2, *S. typhi* Ty2la, or other salmonella strains.

Development of a rotavirus vaccine is a global priority because it is the most common cause of diarrhea in infants in developed and developing nations. Four types of human rotaviruses have been described. Vaccine strains originated from human, rhesus monkey, and bovine sources or were genetically engineered reassortants. Reassortant rhesus strains that express the major human surface antigen (VP7) of each of the four human strains are being tested and have been shown to be safe and immunogenic in field trials. Cold-adapted strains were also shown to be immunogenic. "Nursing" strains derived from infected newborns and the bovine/human virus reassortant (WC3) do not appear to be adequately immunogenic.

Vaccines against enterotoxigenic *E. coli*, the second most common cause of severe diarrhea and the most common cause of travelers' diarrhea, show promise. A live attenuated, nontoxigenic derivative of an enterotoxigenic *E. coli* strain protects volunteers. Vaccine protection correlates with the amount of intestinal IgA directed against colonization factor antigens. A killed vaccine was also produced that induces a satisfactory immune response to the colonization factor antigens as well as to the antitoxin. And finally, synthetic vaccines composed of partial amino-acid sequences from the heat-labile and heat-stable toxins.

Vaccines against shigellosis should contain at least a few of the 30 known serotypes. Necessary components are *Shigella flexneri*, the predominant strain in developed nations, *S. sonnei,* the predominant strain in developing nations, and *S. dysenteriae,* the common epidemic strain. The critical bacterial antigens are the somatic antigens. The ideal vaccine strains should invade the intestinal mucosa, express somatic antigens, and not cause disease. Hybrid strains of *E. coli* and *S. typhi* Ty21a that express *Shigella* somatic antigens have been disappointing because of strain variation or diarrhea in volunteers. Alternatively, certain *S. flexneri* genes have been altered to affect its biosynthetic pathways. The change renders the vaccine strain immunogenic but avirulent. Finally, the lipopolysacchoride antigens in the *Shigella* bacillus have been conjugated to tetanus toxoid as a carrier protein to produce a vaccine that is in Phase 1 trials.

Parasitic Infections

The emergence of chloroquine-resistant *P. falciparum* and the widespread resistance of mosquito vectors to insecticides have added urgency to the need for an effective malaria vaccine because this parasite still causes approximately 1.5 million deaths worldwide each year. Using recombinant DNA techniques, an immunogenic sporozoite protein, the circumsporozoite protein, has been identified and its gene cloned and sequenced.

A synthetic circumsporozoite protein of *P. vivax* expressed in a yeast vector or *P. falciparum* expressed in a baculovirus vector in insect cells has been combined with alum as an adjuvant. The vaccines were poorly immunogenic. Another candidate vaccine is a recombinant protein composed of repeating regions of *P. falciparum* circumsporozoite protein joined to an influenza A nonstructural protein. It is combined with DETOX, a new adjuvant. Despite the stimulation of excellent antibody to the circumsporozoite antigen and the induction of T-cell proliferation, this recombinant vaccine did not provide protection in challenge studies.

Even when the protective efficacy of a sporozoite-derived vaccine is improved, it will only prevent the initial exoerythocytic stage of infection. Because each stage of infection results in a stage-specific immune response, studies are also underway to develop merozoite and gametocyte vaccines.

The most common arthropod-borne viruses are the dengue viruses. Four types are known. Immunity to one type may increase the severity of the illness when infection occurs with another type. Consequently, a vaccine must contain all four types. Live, attenuated mutant vaccines are being tested in initial clinical trials.

Fungal Infections

Progress in developing vaccines against fungal infections has been limited. For example, in a recent trial an experimental coccidioidomycosis formalin-killed spherule vaccine did not prevent clinical disease.

Human Immunodeficiency Virus Infections

The continuing spread of HIV infections throughout the world has elicited an unprecedented response from scientists and health professionals. There is perhaps no other disease for which the need for an effective vaccine is more compelling, nor one that presents such difficult challenges for vaccine development.

A number of different HIV-1 vaccines have been developed and are undergoing Phase 1 clinical trials in human volunteers. Vaccines to prevent HIV-1 infection in seronegative persons consist of recombinant gp 160, recombinant gp 120, a synthetic p 17 peptide, and a live recombinant vaccinia virus expressing gp 160. Vaccines being tested to enhance immunity and delay disease progression in HIV-1-seropositive persons are a recombinant gp 160 vaccine for symptomatic seropositive persons; a gamma irradiated, killed, whole virus vaccine and monoclonal anti-CD4 antibodies in patients with acquired immunodeficiency disease syndrome (AIDS)-related complex; and hyperimmune globulin with high titers of HIV-1 antibody in patients with AIDS.

Problems facing the developers of HIV-1 vaccine are numerous. The first problem is that stimulating neutralizing antibody, which is all that is necessary for measles vaccine and other licensed vaccines, is not sufficient to prevent HIV-1 infection. Antibodies to HIV-1, found in high titers in HIV-infected patients, do not alter disease progression. Preventing the development of the latent virus state, which is not necessary for measles vaccine and other licensed vaccines, will be one of the major challenges to vaccine development. Researchers have not been able to make a vaccine against other viruses, such as herpes simplex virus, that survive in humans in the latent state. In addition, the vaccines commonly used to prevent disease may not prevent subclinical infection.

The second problem in HIV vaccine development is strain composition. This virus undergoes frequent antigenic variation. It will be prudent to find stable portions of the viral genome that elicit protective antibody, appropriate cell-mediated immune responses, or both. The "V3" region in the envelope (*env*) gene that has been studied extensively is hypervariable but may contain some conserved sequences that are being studied.

Lack of a suitable animal model in which to produce AIDS after HIV infection is another concern. Making transgenic animals with the human CD4 receptor may facilitate studies in the absence of a practical animal model.

Selecting appropriate subjects for human vaccine trials is another dilemma, with all of its attendant legal, social, and ethical questions. For example, seronegative patients may not volunteer for a clinical trial for fear of being identified as a member of a high-risk group. A worthwhile vaccine efficacy trial might focus on the interruption of maternal-infant transmission in population groups where the seroprevalence of HIV infection in pregnant women is high.

Unique vaccine immune-response markers must also be identified to distinguish immunity from the vaccine from that from natural infection.

Finally, the end point for considering a vaccine safe and effective must be determined. With an average incubation period of 10 years from the onset of HIV infection to the appearance of AIDS, an effective vaccine must prevent initial infection, prevent the virus from emerging from latency, or significantly delay the appearance of AIDS to be considered effective. Consequently, testing a candidate vaccine may take decades before it can be considered safe and effective.

APPENDIX 1. Immunobiologics and Schedules for Adults*†

Generic Name	Primary Schedule and Booster(s)	Indications	Major Precautions and Contraindications‖	Special Considerations
TOXOIDS				
Tetanus-diphtheria toxoid (Td)	Two doses IM 4 weeks apart, third dose 6–12 months after second dose. Booster recommendations: 1) routine Td every 10 years, OR 2) a single mid-life Td booster at age 50 for persons who have completed the full pediatric series including the teenage/young adult booster	All adults	Pregnancy is not a contraindication; however, waiting until the second trimester of pregnancy to administer tetanus and diphtheria toxoids is reasonable to minimize concern about teratogenicity. History of a neurologic reaction or immediate hypersensitivity reaction after a previous dose. History of severe local reaction (Arthustype) after previous dose; such persons should not be given further routine or emergency doses of Td for 10 years	Tetanus prophylaxis in wound management (summarized in text and in Table 6)
LIVE VIRUS VACCINES				
Measles live virus vaccine	One dose SC. A second dose at least 1 month later, preferably with MMR, for special-risk groups (college students, health care workers, or travelers to areas where measles is endemic)	All adults born after 1956 without documentation of live vaccine on or after first birthday, or physician-diagnosed measles or laboratory evidence of immunity; persons born before 1957 are generally considered to be immune	Pregnancy; immunocompromised persons§; history of anaphylactic reaction following egg ingestion or receipt of neomycin (*see* text)	MMR (measles, mumps, and rubella) is the vaccine of choice if recipients are likely to be susceptible to rubella and/or mumps as well as to measles. Persons vaccinated between 1963 and 1967 with a killed measles vaccine alone, killed vaccine followed by live vaccine, or with a vaccine of unknown type should be revaccinated with live measles virus vaccine

Mumps live virus vaccine	One dose SC; no booster	Pregnancy; immunocompromised persons[‡]; history of anaphylactic reaction after egg ingestion or receipt of neomycin (*see* text)	All adults without documentation of live vaccine on or after first birthdays or physician-diagnosed mumps or laboratory evidence of immunity, particularly young adults who work in or congregate in hospitals, colleges, and on military bases should be vaccinated. It is reasonable to consider persons born before 1957 immune, but there is no contraindication to vaccination of older persons. Susceptible travelers should be vaccinated	MMR is the vaccine of choice if recipients are likely to be susceptible to measles and rubella as well as to mumps
Rubella live virus vaccine	One dose SC; no booster	Pregnancy; immunocompromised persons[‡]; history of anaphylactic reaction after receipt of neomycin	Indicated for adults, both male and female, lacking documentation of live vaccine on or after first birthday or laboratory evidence of immunity, particularly young adults who work or congregate in places such as hospitals and colleges and on military bases. Susceptible travelers should be vaccinated	Women pregnant when vaccinated or who become pregnant within 3 months of vaccination should be counseled on the theoretical risks to the fetus. The risk of rubella vaccine-associated malformations in these women is so small as to be negligible. MMR is the vaccine of choice if recipients are likely to be susceptible to measles or mumps as well as to rubella
Smallpox vaccine (vaccinia virus)		THERE ARE NO INDICATIONS FOR THE USE OF SMALLPOX VACCINE IN THE GENERAL CIVILIAN POPULATION		Laboratory workers working with orthopox viruses or health care workers involved in clinical trials of vaccinia-recombinant vaccines

APPENDIX 1. Immunobiologics and Schedules for Adults*† (continued)

Generic Name	Primary Schedule and Booster(s)	Indications	Major Precautions and Contraindications‖	Special Considerations
Yellow fever live attenuated virus (17D strain)	One dose SC 10 days to 10 years before travel; booster every 10 years	Selected persons traveling or living in areas where yellow fever infection exists	Although specific information is not available concerning adverse effects on the developing fetus, it is prudent on theoretical grounds to avoid vaccinating pregnant women unless the individual must travel to where the risk of yellow fever is high. Immunocompromised persons‡; history of hypersensitivity to egg ingestion	Some countries require a valid International Certificate of Vaccination showing receipt of vaccine. If a pregnant woman is to be vaccinated only to satisfy an international requirement, efforts should be made to obtain a waiver letter
LIVE VIRUS AND INACTIVATED VIRUS VACCINES Enhanced potency inactivated poliovirus vaccine (IPV); oral poliovirus (live) vaccine (OPV)	IPV is preferred for primary vaccination, two doses SC 4 weeks apart, a third dose 6–12 months after second. For adults with a completed primary series and for whom a booster is indicated, either OPV or IPV can be given. If immediate protection is needed, OPV is recommended	Persons traveling to areas where wild poliovirus is epidemic or endemic and certain health care personnel. *See* text for recommendations for incompletely immunized adults and adults in households of children to be immunized	Although no convincing evidence documents adverse effects of either OPV or IPV on the pregnant woman or developing fetus, it is prudent on theoretical grounds to avoid vaccinating pregnant women. However, if immediate protection against poliomyelitis is needed, OPV is recommended. OPV should not be given to immunocompromised family members‡; IPV is recommended in such situations	Although a protective immune response to IPV in the immunocompromised person cannot be ensured, IPV is recommended because the vaccine is safe, and some protection may result from its administration

INACTIVATED VIRUS VACCINES

Vaccine	Dose schedule	Indications	Precautions/contraindications	Comments
Hepatitis B inactivated virus vaccine (HB)	Two doses IM 4 weeks apart, third dose 5 months after second. Alternate schedule for one vaccine: three doses IM 4 weeks apart, fourth dose 10 months after the third	Adults at increased risk of occupational, environmental, social, or family exposure	On the basis of limited data, no apparent risk of adverse effects to the developing fetus exists. Because the vaccine contains only noninfectious hepatitis B surface antigen (HBsAg) particles, the risk should be neglible. Pregnancy should *not* be considered a contraindication to vaccination if the woman is otherwise eligible	The vaccine produces neither therapeutic nor adverse effects on hepatitis B Virus (HBV)-infected persons. Prevaccination serologic screening for susceptibility before vaccination may or may not be cost-effective, depending on the costs of vaccination and testing and on the prevalence of immune persons in the group
Influenza (inactivated whole virus and split virus) vaccine	Annual vaccination with current vaccine. Either whole- or split-virus vaccine may be used	Adults with high-risk conditions, residents of nursing homes or other chronic-care facilities, health care personnel, healthy persons ≥65 years old	History of anaphylactic hypersensitivity to egg ingestion	No evidence exists of maternal or fetal risk when vaccine is given to a pregnant woman because of an underlying high-risk condition. A pregnant woman a with high-risk medical condition should receive influenza vaccine regardless of trimester

APPENDIX 1. Immunobiologics and Schedules for Adults*† (continued)

Generic Name	Primary Schedule and Booster(s)	Indications	Major Precautions and Contraindications‖	Special Considerations
Inactivated Japanese encephalitis (JE) virus vaccine	Three 1-mL doses SC at days 0, 7, and 30. A shortened schedule of 0, 7, and 14 days may be used when necessary. Booster doses may be given after 2 years	NOT recommended for all travelers to Asia. Recommended for those spending at least 1 month in endemic areas during the transmission season, especially if travel will include rural areas	Adverse reactions to JE vaccine manifesting as generalized urticaria and angioedema have occurred within minutes to as long as 2 weeks after vaccination. Vaccinees should be observed for 30 minutes after vaccination and should be advised to have ready access to medical care in the 10 days after receiving vaccine

Persons with a history of urticaria appear to have a greater risk for development of adverse reactions to JE vaccine. This history should be considered when considering the risks and benefits of vaccination for an individual patient.

Vaccination with JE vaccine poses an unknown but theoretical risk to the developing fetus, and the vaccine should not be administered routinely during pregnancy | No data exist on the effect of concurrent administration of other vaccines (except limited data for DTP vaccine), drugs (eg, chloroquine, mefloquine), or biological agents on the safety and immunogenicity of JE vaccine |

Human diploid cell rabies vaccine (HDCV) (inactivated, whole virion); rabies vaccine, adsorbed (RVA)

Pre-exposure prophylaxis: two doses IM or ID 1 week apart, third dose 3 weeks after second.
If exposure continues, booster doses every 2 years, or an antibody titer determined and a booster dose given if titer is inadequate

Postexposure prophylaxis: All postexposure treatment should begin with immediate cleansing of the wound with soap and water

Persons not previously immunized as above: human rabies immune-globulin (HRIG) 20 IU/kg body weight, half infiltrated at bite site if possible, remainder IM; and five doses of HDCV, 1 mL IM, one each on days 0, 3, 7, 14, and 28.

Persons who have previously received postexposure prophylaxis with HDCV, received recommended IM pre-exposure series of HDCV, received recommended ID pre-exposure series of HDCV in the United States, or have a previously documented rabies antibody titer considered adequate: two doses of HDCV, 1 mL IM, one each on days 0 and 3

Veterinarians, animal handlers, certain laboratory workers, and persons living in or visiting countries for more than 1 month where rabies is a constant threat

If there is substantial risk of exposure to rabies, pre-exposure vaccination may be indicated during pregnancy. Corticosteroids and immunosuppressive agents can interfere with the development of active immunity. A history of anaphylactic or Type III hypersensitivity reaction to previous dose of HDCV is a contraindication to further rabies vaccination (*see* text)

Complete pre-exposure prophylaxis does not eliminate the need for additional therapy with rabies vaccine after a rabies exposure. The decision for postexposure use of HDCV depends on the species of biting animal, the circumstances of biting incident and the type of exposure (eg, bite, saliva contamination of wound). The type of and schedule for postexposure prophylaxis depends on the person's previous rabies vaccination status, or the result of a previous or current serologic test for rabies antibody. For postexposure prophylaxis, HDCV should always be administered IM *not* ID

APPENDIX 1. Immunobiologics and Schedules for Adults*† (continued)

Generic Name	Primary Schedule and Booster(s)	Indications	Major Precautions and Contraindications‖	Special Considerations
INACTIVATED BACTERIA VACCINES				
Cholera vaccine	Two 0.5-mL doses SC or IM or two 0.2-mL doses ID 1 week to 1 month apart; booster doses (0.5 mL IM or 0.2 mL ID) every 6 months	Travelers to countries requiring evidence of cholera vaccination for entry. The World Health Organization no longer recommends cholera vaccination for travel to or from cholera-endemic areas	No data exist on the safety of cholera vaccination during pregnancy. Use in pregnancy should reflect actual increased risk. Persons who have had severe local or systemic reactions to a previous dose should not be revaccinated	One dose generally satisfies International Health Regulations. Some countries may require evidence of a complete primary series or a booster dose given within 6 months before arrival. Vaccination should not be considered as an alternative to continued careful selection of foods and water. Ideally, cholera and yellow fever vaccine should be administered at least 3 weeks apart
Haemophilus influenzae type b conjugate vaccine	Dosage for adults has not been determined	May be considered for adults at highest theoretical risk (eg, those with anatomic or functional asplenia, HIV infection)	No data exist on the safety of *H. influenzae* type b vaccination during pregnancy	No efficacy data available; not indicated for adult contacts of children with invasive disease

Meningococcal polysaccharide vaccine (quadrivalent A, C, Y, and W-135)	One dose in volume and route specified by manufacturer. The need for booster doses is unknown	Travelers visiting areas of a country that are recognized as having epidemic meningococcal disease	Pregnancy, unless there is substantial risk of infection	Some countries experiencing epidemic meningococcal vaccine of foreign travelers before arrival
Plague vaccine	Three IM doses: first dose, 1 mL; second dose, 0.2 mL 1 month later; third dose, 0.2 mL 5 months after second; booster doses (0.2 mL) at 1- to 2-year intervals if exposure continues	Selected travelers to countries reporting cases for whom avoidance of rodents and fleas is impossible; all laboratory and field personnel working with *Yersinia pestis* organisms possibly resistant to antimicrobial agents; those engaged in *Y. pestis* aerosol experiments or in field operations in areas with enzootic plague where regular exposure to potentially infected wild rodents, rabbits, or their fleas cannot be prevented	Pregnancy, unless there is substantial and unavoidable risk of exposure; persons with known hypersensitivity to any of the vaccine constituents (*see* manufacturer's label); patients who have had severe local or systemic reactions to a previous dose	Prophylactic antibiotics may be indicated after definite exposure regardless of where the exposed persons have been vaccinated
Pneumococcal polysaccharide vaccine (23 valent)	One dose IM or SC. Revaccination recommended for those at highest risk for fatal pneumococcal infection (eg, splenic dysfunction or asplenia) if ≥6 years elapsed since initial vaccination	Adults who are at increased risk for pneumococcal disease and its complications because of underlying health conditions; all older adults, age ≥65 years	The safety of vaccine in pregnant women has not been evaluated; it should not be given during pregnancy unless the risk of infection is high	Pneumococcal and influenza vaccine can be given simultaneously at separate sites

APPENDIX 1. Immunobiologics and Schedules for Adults*† (continued)

Generic Name	Primary Schedule and Booster(s)	Indications	Major Precautions and Contraindications‖	Special Considerations
INACTIVATED BATERIA AND LIVE BACTERIA VACCINES				
Typhoid vaccine, SC, and oral	Two 0.5-mL doses SC 4 or more weeks apart; booster dose 0.5 mL SC or 0.1 mL ID every 3 years if exposure continues. Four oral doses on alternate days. The manufacturer recommends revaccination with the entire four-dose series every 5 years	Travelers to areas where a recognized risk of exposure to typhoid exists	Severe local or systemic reaction to a previous dose. Acetone-killed and -dried vaccines should not be given ID	Vaccination should not be considered as an alternative to continued careful selection of foods and water
LIVE BACTERIA VACCINE				
Bacille Calmette-Guérin (BCG)	One dose ID or SC (see package label)	BCG vaccination is no longer recommended for adults at high risk for tuberculosis in the United States. BCG vaccination may be considered for infants and children who have negative skin test results to 5 units of tuberculin and who cannot be given isoniazid preventive therapy but have close contact with untreated or ineffectively treated active tuberculosis patients or who belong to groups with excessive rates of new infection in which other control measures have not been successful	Pregnancy, unless there is unavoidable exposure to infectious tuberculosis; immunocompromised patients‡	In the United States, tuberculosis control efforts are directed toward early identification, treatment of cases, and preventive therapy with isoniazid

IMMUNE GLOBULINS

	Dosage	Indication/Population	Comments
Cytomegalovirus immune globulin (intravenous)	Bone marrow transplant recipients: 1 g/kg weekly; kidney transplant recipients: 150 mg/kg initially, then 50-100 mg/kg every 2 weeks	As prophylaxis for bone marrow and kidney transplant recipients	Prophylaxis must be continued for 3–4 months to be effective
Immune globulin (IG)	Hepatitis A prophylaxis: Before exposure — One IM dose of 0.02 mL/kg for anticipated risk of 3 months; IM dose of 0.06 mL/kg for anticipated risk of ≥3 months; repeat at 4- to 6-month intervals if exposure continues	Nonimmune persons traveling to developing countries	For travelers, IG is not an alternative to careful selection of foods and water. Frequent travelers should be tested for hepatitis A antibody. Immune globulin can interfere with the antibody response to parenterally administered live virus vaccines. IG is not indicated for persons with antibody to hepatitis A
	After exposure—One IM dose of 0.02 mL/kg given within 2 weeks of exposure	Household and sexual contacts of persons with hepatitis A; staff, attendees, and parents of diapered attendees in daycare center outbreaks	
	Measles prophylaxis: 0.25 mL/kg IM (maximum, 15 mL) given within 6 days after exposure	Exposed susceptible contacts of measles cases	IG should *not* be used to control measles / IG given within 6 days after exposure can prevent or modify measles. Recipients of IG for measles prophylaxis should receive live measles vaccine 5 months later
Intravenous immune globulin (IVIG)	150 mg/kg every 3 to 4 weeks. Patient requirements vary considerably, and dosage schedules must be individualized	Specific and combined immunodeficiency diseases, malignancies with antibody deficiencies, burns, bone marrow transplantation, and nephrotic syndrome	Anaphylactic hypersensitivity reactions can occur, especially in IgA-deficient patients / Therapy should be guided by clinical observation and serial determination of serum IgG levels. IVIG cannot transmit HIV or hepatitis B virus infections

APPENDIX 1.   Immunobiologics and Schedules for Adults*† (continued)

Generic Name	Primary Schedule and Booster(s)	Indications	Major Precautions and Contraindications‖	Special Considerations
Hepatitis B immune globulin (HBIG)	0.06 mL/kg IM as soon as possible after exposure (with HB vaccine started at a different site); a second dose of HBIG should be given 1 month later if the HB vaccine series has not been started	After percutaneous or mucous membrane exposures to blood known to be HBsAg positive (within 7 days); after sexual exposure to a person with acute HBV or an HBV carrier (within 14 days); at birth for infants born of HBsAg-positive mothers		Hepatitis B vaccine should also be given if the patient will be at continued risk of exposure to HB (for example, health care workers, infants born to a mother who is an HBsAg carrier)
Tetanus immune globulin (TIG)	250 units IM	Part of management of nonclean, nonminor wound in a person with unknown tetanus toxoid status, with fewer than two previous doses, or with two previous doses and a wound more than 24 hours old		
Rabies immune globulin, human (HRIG)	20 IU/kg, up to one half infiltrated around wound, remained IM	Part of management of rabies exposure in persons lacking a history of recommended preexposure or postexposure prophylaxis with rabies vaccine or a recently documented neutralizing antibody response to previous rabies vaccination		Although it is preferable to give HRIG with the first dose of vaccine, it can be given as long as 8 days after vaccination

| Varicella zoster immune globulin (VZIG) | Persons ≤50 kg: 125 units/10 kg IM; persons >50 kg: 625 units[§] | Immunocompromised patients known or likely to be susceptible with close and prolonged exposure to a household contact or to an infectious hospital staff member or hospital roommate; perinatal prophylaxis and treatment of mothers and prophylaxis of infants born to mothers with varicella. | VZIG is not indicated for prophylaxis or therapy of healthy adults who are exposed to or who develop varicella. Also, it is not indicated for treatment of herpes zoster. An acceptable alternative to VZIG phrophylaxis is to treat varicella, if it occurs, with high-dose intravenous acyclovir |

---

* Several other vaccines, toxoids, and immune globulins are licensed and available. These are noted in Appendix 2. In addition, the following antitoxins are licensed and available: a) botulism antitoxin, trivalent (ABE) equine (distributed by Centers for Disease Control and Prevention [CDC] only); b) tetanus antitoxin (equine); and c) diphtheria antitoxin (distributed by CDC only). IM = intramuscularly; SC = subcutaneously.

† Several vaccines and toxoids have "Investigation of New Drug" (IND) status and are available only through the U.S. Army Research Institute for Infectious Diseases (telephone 301-663-2403). These are a) eastern equine encephalitis (EEE) vaccine; b) western equine encephalitis (WEE) vaccine; c) Venezuelan equine encephalitis (VEE) vaccine; and d) tularemia vaccine. Pentavalant (ABCDE) botulinum toxoid is available only through CDC's Drug Service.

‡ Persons immunocompromised because of immune deficiency diseases, HIV infection (who should primarily not receive OPV and yellow fever vaccines, *see* text), leukemia, lymphoma, or generalized malignancy or who are immunosuppressed as a result of therapy with corticosteroids, alkylating drugs, antimetabolites, or radiation.

§ Some experts recommend 125 units/10 kg regardless of total body weight.

‖ When any vaccine or toxoid is indicated during pregnancy, waiting until the second or third trimester, when possible, is a reasonable precaution that minimizes concern about teratogenicity.

NOTE: Refer to text on specific vaccines, toxoids, or immune globulin preparations for further details on clinical effectiveness, indications, administration, adverse reactions, precautions, contraindications, and revaccination. Refer to package inserts for current information on dosages and routes of administration.

Source: National Immunization Program, Centers for Disease Control and Prevention, May 1993.

APPENDIX 2. Immunobiologic Products, Dates Licensed, Manufacturers, and Telephone Numbers

Product	Date Licensed	Manufacturer/Distributor	Telephone Number
Adenovirus Vaccine			
Adenovirus, Live, Oral, Type 4	07/01/80	Wyeth-Ayerst Laboratories, Inc*	800-321-2304
Adenovirus, Live, Oral, Type 7	07/01/80	Wyeth-Ayerst Laboratories, Inc*	800-321-2304
Anthrax Vaccine			
Anthrax Vaccine Adsorbed	11/04/70	Michigan Department of Public Health†	517-335-8119
Bacille Calmette-Guérin Vaccine			
BCG Vaccine		Organon Teknika Corporation	800-323-6442
Cholera Vaccine			
Cholera Vaccine	07/16/52	Wyeth-Ayerst Laboratories, Inc	800-321-2304
Diphtheria Antitoxin			
Purified, Concentrated Globulin-EQUINE	01/03/78	Connaught Laboratories, Inc	800-822-2463
Diphtheria and Tetanus Toxoids Adsorbed			
Diphtheria and Tetanus Toxoids Adsorbed (Pediatric)	9/18/84	Connaught Laboratories, Inc.	800-822-2463
Diphtheria and Tetanus Toxoids Adsorbed (Purogenated for Pediatric Use)	3/22/54	Lederle Laboratories	914-732-5000
Diphtheria and Tetanus Toxoids Adsorbed (Pediatric)	5/23/50	Massachusetts Public Health Biologic Laboratories	617-522-3700
Diphtheria and Tetanus Toxoids Adsorbed (Pediatric)	5/11/51	Michigan Department of Public Health†	517-335-8119
Diphtheria and Tetanus Toxoids Adsorbed (Pediatric)		Wyeth-Ayerst Laboratories, Inc	800-321-2304
Diphtheria and Tetanus Toxoids and Pertussis Vaccine Adsorbed			
Diphtheria and Tetanus Toxoids and Pertussis Vaccine Adsorbed	01/03/78	Connaught Laboratories, Inc	800-822-2463
Tri Immunol	07/24/70	Lederle Laboratories	914-732-5000

Diphtheria and Tetanus Toxoids and Pertussis Vaccine		
Adsorbed	07/27/70	Massachusetts Public Health Biologic Laboratories	617-522-3700
Diphtheria and Tetanus Toxoids and Pertussis Vaccine			
Adsorbed[‡]	08-27-70	Michigan Department of Public Health[†§]	517-335-8119
Diphtheria and Tetanus Toxoids and Accelluar Pertussis Vaccine Adsorbed			
Tripedia	08/21/92	Connaught Laboratories, Inc	800-822-2463
Acelimune	12/17/91	Lederle Laboratories	800-533-3753
Diphtheria and Tetanus Toxoids and Pertussis Vaccine Adsorbed and *Haemophilus influenzae* type b conjugate Vaccine			
Tetraimune	03/30/93	Lederle-Praxis Biologicals	800-533-3753
ActHIB (may be reconstituted		Connaught Laboratories, Inc	800-822-2463
with Connaught's DTP vaccine)			
***Haemophilus influenzae* type b Vaccine (conjugate)**			
ProHIBiT	12/22/87	Connaught Laboratories, Inc	800-822-2463
Hibtiter	12/21/88	Lederle-Praxis Biologicals	800-533-3753
Pedvax HiB	12/20/89	Merck Sharp & Dohme	215-652-5000
ActHIB	03/30/93	Connaught Laboratories, Inc	800-822-2463
Hepatitis B Immune Globulin (Human)			
H-BIG	06/15/77	Abbott Laboratories	800-323-9100
Hep-B-Gammagee	12/06/78	Merck Sharp & Dohme	215-652-5000
Hyper-Hep	09/23/77	Miles, Inc	800-288-8371
Hepatitis B Vaccine (Recombinant)			
Recombivax HB	07/23/86	Merck Sharp & Dohme	215-652-5000
Engerix-B	08/28/89	SmithKline Beecham	215-751-5231
Immune Globulin Intravenous (Human)			
Gammar-IV	10/13/88	Armour Pharmaceutical Company	800-727-6737
Gammagard	02/18/86	Baxter Healthcare Corporation	800-423-2090

APPENDIX 2. Immunobiologic Products, Dates Licensed, Manufacturers, and Telephone Numbers (continued)

Product	Date Licensed	Manufacturer/Distributor	Telephone Number
Sandoglobulin	06/07/84	Central Laboratory Blood Transfusion Service, Swiss Red Cross‖	201-503-7500
Gamimune	09/11/81	Miles, Inc	800-288-8371
IVEEGAM		Immuno-US	313-652-7872
Venoglobulin-1		Alpha Therapeutics	800-421-0008
Immune Globulin (Human)			
Gammar	05/17/49	Armour Pharmaceutical Company	800-727-6737
Immune Globulin (Human)	09/08/43	Massachusetts Public Health Biologic Laboratories§	617-522-3700
Immune Globulin (Human)	12/22/50	Michigan Department of Public Health†§	517-335-8119
Gamastan	01/11/44	Miles, Inc.	800-288-8371
Immune Globulin (Human)	06/01/73	New York Blood Center, Inc	212-570-3137
Influenza Virus Vaccine			
Whole Virion Fluzone	01/03/73	Connaught Laboratories, Inc	800-822-2463
Split Virion Fluzone	01/03/73	Connaught Laboratories, Inc	800-822-2463
Split Virion Fluogen	11/26/45	Parke-Davis	201-540-2000
Influenza Virus Vaccine Trivalent Types A and B (Chromatograph), Subvirion Type	12/13/61	Wyeth-Ayerst Laboratories, Inc	800-321-2304
Split Virion Fluimune	07/11/89	Lederle Laboratories	800-533-3753
Japanese Encephalitis Virus Vaccine, Inactivated			
JE-VAX		Connaught Laboratories, Inc. (U.S. distributor for Biken of Japan)	800-822-2463
Measles Vaccine			
Attenuvax	03/21/63	Merck Sharp & Dohme	215-652-5000

Vaccine / Product	Date	Manufacturer	Phone
Measles and Rubella			
M-R-VAXII	04/22/71	Merck Sharp & Dohme	215-652-5000
Measles, Mumps, and Rubella Vaccine			
MMRII	04/22/71	Merck Sharp & Dohme	215-652-5000
Meningococcal Polysaccharide Vaccine			
Menomune-A/C/Y/W-135	01/03/78	Connaught Laboratories, Inc	800-822-2463
Mumps Vaccine			
Mumpsvax	12/28/67	Merck Sharp & Dohme	215-652-5000
Pertussis Vaccine Adsorbed			
Pertussis Vaccine Adsorbed	10/12/67	Michigan Department of Public Health[†§]	517-335-8119
Plague Vaccine			
Plague Vaccine	05/14/42	Miles, Inc	800-288-8371
Pneumococcal Polysaccharide Vaccine, Polyvalent			
Pnu-Imune 23	08/15/79	Lederle Laboratories	914-732-5000
Pneumovax 23	11/21/77	Merck Sharp & Dohme	215-652-5000
Poliovirus Vaccine, Enhanced Potency Inactivated			
Poliovax, Human Diploid Cell Vaccine	01/20/87	Connaught Laboratories, Inc	800-822-2463
Poliovirus Vaccine, Live Oral			
Orimune	06/25/63	Lederle Laboratories	914-732-5000
Rabies Immune Globulin (Human)			
Imogam	04/27/84	Connaught Laboratories, Inc	800-822-2463
Hyperab	06/12/74	Miles, Inc	800-288-8371
Rabies Vaccine			
Imovax, Human Diploid Cell Vaccine	06/09/80	Connaught Laboratories, Inc	800-822-2463

APPENDIX 2. Immunobiologic Products, Dates Licensed, Manufacturers, and Telephone Numbers (continued)

Product	Date Licensed	Manufacturer/Distributor	Telephone Number
Rabies Vaccine, Adsorbed	03/18/88	Michigan Department of Public Health[†]	517-335-8119
Rubella and Mumps Vaccine			
Biavax II	08/30/70	Merck Sharp & Dohme	215-652-5000
Rubella Virus Vaccine			
Meruvax II	06/09/69	Merck Sharp & Dohme	215-652-5000
Tetanus and Diphtheria Toxoids Adsorbed			
Tetanus and Diphtheria Toxoids Adsorbed (For Adult Use)	01/03/78	Connaught Laboratories, Inc	800-822-2463
Tetanus and Diphtheria Toxoids Adsorbed (For Adult Use) (Purogenated Parenteral)	07/29/70	Lederle Laboratories	914-732-5000
Tetanus and Diphtheria Toxoids Adsorbed (For Adult Use)	07/27/70	Massachusetts Public Health Biologic Laboratories	617-522-3700
Tetanus and Diphtheria Toxoids Adsorbed (For Adult Use) [Aluminum Phosphate, Ultrafined]	09/11/70	Wyeth-Ayerst Laboratories, Inc	800-321-2304
Tetanus Immune Globulin (Human)			
Tetanus Immune Globulin (Human)	05/06/68	Massachusetts Public Health Biologic Laboratories[§]	617-522-3700
Hypertet	08/15/78	Miles, Inc	800-288-8371
Tetanus Toxoid Adsorbed			
Tetanus Toxoid Adsorbed	01/03/78	Connaught Laboratories, Inc	800-822-2463
Tetanus Toxoid Adsorbed (Purogenated, Aluminum Phosphate Adsorbed)	07/29/70	Lederle Laboratories	914-732-5000
Tetanus Toxoid Adsorbed	07/27/70	Massachusetts Public Health Biologic Laboratories[§]	617-522-3700
Tetanus Toxoid Adsorbed	08/27/70	Michigan Department of Public Health[†§]	517-335-8119
Tetanus Toxoid Adsorbed (Aluminum Phosphate Adsorbed, Ultrafined)	09/11/70	Wyeth-Ayerst Laboratories, Inc	800-321-2304

Tetanus Toxoid Fluid

Tetanus Toxoid	01/14/43	Connaught Laboratories, Inc	800-822-2463
Tetanus Toxoid (Fluid, Purified, Ultrafined)	05/19/44	Wyeth-Ayerst Laboratories, Inc	800-321-2304

Typhoid Vaccine

Typhoid Vaccine	07/16/52	Wyeth-Ayerst Laboratories, Inc	800-321-2304
Typhoid Vaccine, live oral Ty21a Vivotif Berna	01/08/90	Swiss Serum and Vaccine Institute	800-533-5899

Vaccinia Immune Globulin (Human)

Vaccinia Immune Globulin (Human)	12/31/68	None (CDC and Department of Defense stockpiles only)	404-639-3670

Vaccinia Vaccine

Vaccinia Vaccine	1903	None (CDC and Department of Defense stockpiles only)	404-639-3670

Varicella Zoster Immune Globulin (Human)

Varicella Zoster Immune Globulin (Human)	12/23/80	Massachusetts Public Health Biologic Laboratories¶	617-522-3700

Yellow Fever Vaccine

Live, 17D Virus, ALV-Free YF-VAX	01/03/78	Connaught Laboratories, Inc	800-822-2463

* Available only to the United States Armed Forces.

† Outside Michigan sold only to providers who will sign a "hold harmless" agreement.

‡ The acetone-killed and -dried form of the vaccine is available only to the United States Armed Forces.

§ Limited distribution to public health agencies only.

‖ Distributed in the United States by Sandoz Pharmaceuticals, East Hanover, New Jersey.

¶ Varicella zoster immune globulin is available from selected blood banks in various locations in the United States. For a listing, consult MMWR 1991;40 (No.RR-12):89-94.

Note: In the preparation of this appendix, every effort was made to ensure its completeness and accuracy. It was compiled from information obtained from manufacturers, the Division of Product Certification, Food and Drug Administration, and the Physicians Desk Reference, 47th edition, 1993. To the best of our knowledge, it is an accurate and complete listing as of 1 December 1993. However, omissions and errors may have occurred inadvertently. The appendix is intended to be a resource and does not replace the provider's obligation to remain current on the availability of vaccines, toxoids, and immune globulins.

Appendix 3

Recommendations of the Advisory Committee on Immunization Practices (ACIP)

Recommendation	*MMWR* Citation
General recommendations on immunization	1994;43(RR-1):1-39
Adult immunization	1991;40(RR-12):1–94
Altered immunocompetence	1993;42(RR-4):1–18
Bacille Calmette-Guérin	1988;37:663–4, 669–75
Cholera	1988;37:617–24
Diphtheria, tetanus, and pertussis	1991;40(RR-10):1–28
Pertussis, acellular (supplementary statements)	1992;41:(RR-1):1–10 1992;41:(RR-15):1–5
Haemophilus influenzae type b	1991;40(RR-1):1–7 1993;42(RR-13):1–15
Hepatitis, viral	1990;39(RR-2):1–26 1991;40(RR-13):1–25
Influenza*	1993;42(RR-6):1–14
Japanese encephalitis	1993;42(RR-1):1–15
Measles	1989;38:(S9):1–18
Meningococcal polysaccharide vaccine	1985;34:255–9
Mumps	1989;38:388–92, 397–400
Plague	1982;31:301–4
Pneumococcal	1989;38:64–8, 73–6
Poliomyelitis	1982;31:22–6,31–4
Poliomyelitis, enhanced potency inactivated vaccine	1987;36:795–8
Rabies	1991;40(RR-3):1–19
Rubella	1990;39(RR-15):1–18
Typhoid	1990;39(RR-10):1–5
Vaccinia (smallpox)	1991;40(RR-14):1–10
Varicella zoster immune globulin	1984;33:84–90,95–100
Yellow fever	1990;39(RR-6):1–6

* Each year influenza vaccine recommendations are reviewed and amended to reflect updated information on influenza activity in the United States for the preceding influenza season and to provide information on the vaccine available for the upcoming influenza season. These recommendations are published in the *Mortality and Morbidity Weekly Report* (*MMWR*) annually, usually in May or June.

APPENDIX 4

State Immunization Requirements* Applicable to Some or All Schools[†] (Grades K–12) and to Some or All Colleges/Universities[‡]

State	Diphtheria		Tetanus		Pertussis		Measles		Mumps		Rubella		Polio	
	Schools	Colleges	Schools	Colleges	Schools	Colleges	Schools	Colleges	Schools	Colleges	Schools	Colleges	Schools	Colleges
Alabama	K-12		K-12		K-6 yrs		K-12		K-12		K-12		K-12	
Alaska	K-12		K-12		K-6 yrs		K-12		Not Required	Not Required	K-12		K-12	
Arizona	K-12		K-12		K-12		K-12	S[§]	K-12		K-12		K-12	
Arkansas	K-12		K-12		K-6 yrs		K-12	U[§]	Not Required	Not Required	K-12	U[§]	K-12	
California	K-12		K-12		K-6 yrs		K-12	S[‖]	K-12		K-12	S[‖]	K-12	
Colorado	K-12		K-12		K-6 yrs		K-12		K-12		K-12		K-12	
Connecticut	K-12		K-12		K-6 yrs		K-12	U[§]	K-12		K-12	U[§]	K-12	
Delaware	K-12		K-12		K-6 yrs		K-12	U[§]	K-12		K-12		K-12	
Dist. of Col.	K-12	U[§]	K-12	U[§]	K-6 yrs		K-12	U[§]	K-12	U[§]	K-12	U[§]	K-12	U[§]
Florida	K-12		K-12		K-6 yrs		K-12	S[‖]	K-12	S[‖]	K-12	S[‖]	K-12	
Georgia	K-12		K-12		K-6 yrs		K-12	S[‖]	K-12	S[‖]	K-12	S[‖]	K-12	
Hawaii	K-12		K-12		K-6 yrs	Not Required	K-12		K-12		K-12		K-12	
Idaho	K-5		K-5		Not Required		K-5		K-5		K-5		K-5	
Illinois	K-12	S[‖]	K-12	S[‖]	K-12		K-12	S[‖]	K-12	S[‖]	K-12	S[‖]	K-12	S[‖]
Indiana	K-12		K-12		K-6 yrs		K-12		K-7		K-12		K-12	

State Immunization Requirements* Applicable to Some or All Schools† (Grades K-12) and to Some or All Colleges/Universities‡

State	Diphtheria Schools	Diphtheria Colleges	Tetanus Schools	Tetanus Colleges	Pertussis Schools	Pertussis Colleges	Measles Schools	Measles Colleges	Mumps Schools	Mumps Colleges	Rubella Schools	Rubella Colleges	Polio Schools	Polio Colleges
Iowa	K-12		K-12		K-6 yrs		K-12	S‖	Not Required	Not Required	K-12	S‖	K-12	
Kansas	K-12		K-12		K-6 yrs		K-12		K-12	K-12	K-12		K-12	
Kentucky	K-12		K-12		Not Required	Not Required	K-12		Not Required	Not Required	K-12		K-12	
Louisiana	New Enterers	New Enterers	New Enterers	New Enterers	New Enterers	New Enterers	New Enterers	New Enterers	New Enterers	New Enterers	New Enterers	New Enterers	New Enterers	
Maine	K-12	U§	K-12	U§	Not Required	Not Required	K-12	U§	K-12	U§	K-12	U§	K-12	
Maryland	K-12		K-12		K-6 yrs		K-12		Not Required	Not Required	K-12		K-12	
Massachusetts	K-12	U§	K-12	U§	K-6 yrs		K-12	U§	K-12		K-12	U§	K-12	
Michigan	New Enterers	New Enterers	New Enterers	New Enterers	New Enterers	New Enterers	New Enterers	New Enterers	New Enterers	New Enterers	New Enterers	New Enterers	New Enterers	
Minnesota	K-12	U§	K-12	U§	K-6 yrs		K-12	U§	K-12	U§	K-12	U§	K-12	
Mississippi	K-12		K-12		K-6 yrs		K-12	S‖	New Enterers		K-12	S‖	K-12	
Missouri	K-12		K-12	U§	Not Required	Not Required	K-12	U§	Not Required	Not Required	K-12	U§	K-12	
Montana	K-12		K-12		K-12		K-12		K-13		K-12		K-12	
Nebraska	K-12		K-12	U§	K-6 yrs		K-12		K-12		K-12		K-12	
Nevada	K-12		K-12	U§	K-6 yrs		K-12	U§	K-12	U§	K-12	U§	K-12	
New Hampshire	K-12		K-12		K-6 yrs		K-12		K-12		K-12		K-12	
New Jersey	K-12		K-12		K-6 yrs		K-12	U§	K-12	U§	K-12	U§	K-12	
New Mexico	K-12		K-12		K-6 yrs		K-12		Not Required	Not Required	K-12		K-12	
New York	K-12		Not Required	Not Required	Not Required	Not Required	K-12	U§	K-12		K-12	U§	K-12	

State														
North Carolina	K-12	U§	K-12	U§	K-6 yrs	U§	K-12	U§	K-12	U§	K-12	U§	K-12	U§
North Dakota	K-12		K-12		K-6 yrs		K-12	S‖	K-12	S‖	K-12	S‖	K-12	S‖
Ohio	K-12		K-12		K-6 yrs		K-12		K-12		K-12		K-12	
Oklahoma	K-12		K-12		K-6 yrs		K-12		K-4		K-12		K-12	
Oregon	K-12		K-12		Not Required		K-12		K-11		K-12		K-12	
Pennsylvania	K-12		K-12		Not Required		K-12		K-12		K-12		K-12	
Puerto Rico	K-12		K-12		K-6 yrs		K-12	U§	K-12	U§	K-12	U§	K-12	U§
Rhode Island	K-12		K-12		K-6 yrs		K-12	U§	K-12	U§	K-12	U§	K-12	
South Carolina	K-12		K-12		K-6 yrs		K-12		K-12		K-12		K-12	
South Dakota	K-12	S‖	K-12	S‖	K-6 yrs	S‖	K-12	S‖	K-12	S‖	K-12	S‖	K-12	S‖
Tennessee	K-12		K-12		K-6 yrs		K-12	S‖	K-13		K-12		K-12	
Texas	K-12		K-12		Not Required		K-12		K-12		K-12		K-12	
Utah	K-12		K-12		K-6 yrs		K-12		K-12		K-12		K-12	
Vermont	K-12		K-12		K-6 yrs		K-12		Not Required		K-12		K-12	
Virginia	K-12	S‖	K-12	S‖	K-6 yrs	S‖	K-12	S‖	K-12	S‖	K-12	S‖	K-12	S‖
Washington	K-12		K-12		Not Required		K-12		K-1		K-12		K-12	
West Virginia	K-12		K-12		K-6		New Enterers	S‖	Not Required	S‖	K-12	S‖	K-12	S‖
Wisconsin	K-12		K-12		K-6 yrs		K-12		K-12		K-12		K-12	
Wyoming	K-12		K-12		K-6 yrs		K-12	S‖	K-12	S‖	K-12	S‖	K-12	S‖

* State immunization requirements may be by statute and/or rule or regulation. In addition, for colleges and universities, requirements may be established by a statewide governing body (for example, a board of regents).

† This table represents the most current information available on school immunization requirements as of 1 June 1993. Periodically, states may change their school requirements by adding or deleting certain vaccines or by extending the grades to which these requirements apply. To obtain updated information or clarify any questions regarding school immunization requirements, contact school officials or public health officials in the state or locality where the school in question is located.

‡ This table represents the most current information available on college and university immunization requirements as of 1 June 1993. Subsequently, some states may have established college and university immunization requirements. Many institutions not covered by state requirements have elected to establish their own. To obtain updated information or clarify any questions regarding specific requirements, contact college and university or state public health officials in the state where the institution in question is located.

§ Universal: state immunization requirements extend to **all** institutions of higher learning.

‖ Selected: state immunization requirements apply only to certain categories of institutions (for example, all public colleges and universities or all 4-year colleges and universities).

Appendix 5

State and Territorial Health Departments

Alabama
Department of Public Health
State Office Building
Montgomery, AL 36130-1701
205-261-5052

Alaska
Department of Health & Social
    Services
Alaska Office Building
Pouch H 06
Juneau, AK 99811
907-465-3090

Arizona
Department of Health Services
1740 W Adams Street
Phoenix, AZ 85007
602-255-1024

Arkansas
Department of Health
4815 W Markham Street
Little Rock, AR 72205-3867
501-661-2000

California
Department of Health Services
714 P Street, Room 1253
Sacramento, CA 95814
916-445-1248

Colorado
Department of Health
4300 Cherry Creek Drive South
Denver, CO 80222-1530
303-692-2000

Connecticut
State Department of Health
    Services
150 Washington Street
Hartford, CT 06106
203-566-2279

Delaware
Department of Health & Social
    Services
Division of Public Health
Jesse Cooper Building
Capitol Square
Dover, DE 19901
302-736-4701

District of Columbia
Department of Human Services
Commission of Public Health
1660 L Street, NW
Washington, DC 20036
202-673-7700

Florida

Department of Health &
　Rehabilitative Services
1323 Winewood Boulevard, #115
Tallahassee, FL 32399-0700
904-487-2705

Georgia

Department of Human Resources
Division of Public Health
878 Peachtree Street, NE
Atlanta, GA 30309
404-894-7505

Hawaii

Department of Health
Kiau Hale, PO Box 3378
Honolulu, HI 96801
808-548-6505

Idaho

Department of Health & Welfare
Division of Health
450 W State
Boise, ID 83720
208-334-5930

Illinois

Department of Public Health
535 W Jefferson Street
Springfield, IL 62761
217-782-4977

Indiana

State Board of Health
1330 W Michigan Street
Box 1964
Indianapolis, IN 46206
317-633-8400

Iowa

Department of Health
Lucas State Office Building
Des Moines, IA 50319
515-281-5605

Kansas

State Department of Health &
　Environment
900 SW Jackson, Room 620
Topeka, KS 66612
913-296-1500

Kentucky

Cabinet for Human Resources
Department of Health Services
275 E Main Street
Frankfort, KY 40621
502-564-3970

Louisiana

Department of Health & Human
　Resources
Office of Health Services &
　Environmental Quality
325 Loyola Avenue
PO Box 60630
New Orleans, LA 70160
504-568-5052

Maine

Department of Human Services
Bureau of Health
151 Capital Street
Augusta, ME 04333
207-287-3201

Maryland

State Department of Health &
    Mental Hygiene
201 W Preston Street
Baltimore, MD 21201
301-225-6500

Massachusetts

Department of Public Health
150 Tremont Street
Boston, MA 02111
617-727-2700

Michigan

Department of Public Health
3500 N Logan Street
Box 30035
Lansing, MI 48909
517-335-8024

Minnesota

Department of Health
717 Delaware Street, SE
Minneapolis, MN 55440
612-623-5100

Mississippi

State Department of Health
2423 N State Street
Box 1700
Jackson, MS 39215
601-960-7634

Missouri

Department of Health
1738 E Elm
Box 570
Jefferson City, MO 65102
314-751-6400

Montana

State Department of Health &
    Environmental Sciences
Cogswell Building
PO Box 200901
Helena, MT 59620-0901
406-444-2544

Nebraska

State Department of Health
301 Centennial Mall South
Lincoln, NE 68509
402-471-2133

Nevada

State Department of Human
    Resources
Division of Health
Capitol Complex
505 E King Street
Carson City, NV 89710
702-885-4740

New Hampshire

State Department of Health &
    Welfare
Division of Public Health
Health & Welfare Building
Hazen Drive
Concord, NH 03301
603-271-4477

New Jersey

State Department of Health
CN 360
John Fitch Plaza
Trenton, NJ 08625
609-292-7837

New Mexico

Department of Health
PO Box 26110
Santa Fe, NM 87502-6110
505-827-2613

New York

State Department of Health
Corning Tower
Empire State Plaza
Albany, NY 12237
518-474-7354

North Carolina

Department of Human Resources
Division of Health Services
PO Box 27687
Raleigh, NC 27611
919-733-7752

North Dakota

State Department of Health
State Capitol Building
Bismarck, ND 58505
701-224-2372

Ohio

Department of Health
246 N High Street
7th Floor
Columbus, OH 43266-0588
614-466-2253

Oklahoma

State Department of Health
1000 NE 10th
Oklahoma City, OK 73117

Oregon

State Health Division
800 NE Oregon Street
Portland, OR 97232
503-731-4020

Pennsylvania

State Department of Health
PO Box 90
Harrisburg, PA 17108
717-787-6436

Rhode Island

Department of Health
3 Capitol Hill
Providence, RI 02908
401-277-2231

South Carolina

Department of Health &
    Environmental Control
J Marion Sims Building
2600 Bull Street
Columbia, SC 29201
803-734-4880

South Dakota

State Department of Health
Joe Foss Building
523 E Capitol Avenue
Pierre, SD 57501
605-773-3361

Tennessee

Department of Health
Cordell Hull Building
Room 344
Nashville, TN 37247-0101
615-741-3111

Texas

Department of Health
1100 W 49th Street
Austin, TX 78756
512-458-7375

Utah

Department of Health
PO Box 16700
Salt Lake City, UT 84116-0700
801-538-6111

Vermont

Department of Health
108 Cherry Street
PO Box 70
Burlington, VT 05402
802-863-7200

Virginia

State Department of Health
The James Madison Building
109 Governor Street
Richmond, VA 23219
804-786-3561

Washington

Department of Health
PO Box 47890
Olympia, WA 98504-7890
206-753-5871

West Virginia

State Department of Health
1800 Washington Street
Charleston, WV 25305
304-348-2971

Wisconsin

Department of Health & Social
  Services
Division of Health
One W Wilson Street

Box 309
Madison, WI 53701-0309
608-266-1511

Wyoming

Department of Health & Social
  Services
Division of Health & Medical
  Services
Hathaway Building
Cheyenne, WY 82002
307-777-7121

American Samoa

Department of Health
LBJ Tropical Medical Center
Pago Pago, A. Samoa 96799

Micronesia

Department of Human Resources
PO Box PS70
Palikir, Pohnpei FM 96941

Guam

Department of Public Health
PO Box 2816
Agana, Guam 96901

Puerto Rico

Department of Health
Building A, Call Box 70184
San Juan, PR 00936

Mariana Islands

Department of Health
PO Box 409CK
Saipan, CM 96950

Virgin Islands

Department of Health
PO Box 7309, Charlotte Amalle
St. Thomas, VI 00801

APPENDIX 6

Sources for Vaccine Information

Information on specific vaccines can be obtained by telephoning
Public Inquiries, Centers for Disease Control and Prevention
404-639-3534

Department of Health and Human Services
U.S. Public Health Service
Centers for Disease Control and Prevention
Atlanta, GA 30333
404-639-3311

Center for Biologics Evaluation and Research
Food and Drug Administration
8800 Rockville Pike
Bethesda, MD 20892
301-496-3556

Expanded Program on Immunization
Pan American Health Organization
525 23rd Street, NW
Washington, DC 20037
202-861-3247

Biologic Products Program
Michigan Department of Public Health
3500 North Logan
Lansing, MI 48909
517-335-8120

U.S. Army Medical Research Institute for Infectious Diseases
Fort Detrick
Frederick, MD 21701
301-663-8000

Report of the Committee on Infectious Diseases (The Red Book)
American Academy of Pediatrics
P.O. Box 927
Elk Grove Village, IL 60009-0927
800-433-9016

Control of Communicable Diseases in Man (The Manual)
American Public Health Association
1015 Fifteenth Street, NW
Washington, DC 20005
202-789-5600

Health Information for International Travel (The Yellow Book)
Superintendent of Documents
U.S. Government Printing Office
Washington, DC 20402
202-783-3238

Health Information for International Travel
World Health Organization
1211 Geneva 27, Suite 7
Switzerland

Appendix 7

Patient Immunization Record

Patient Name: _____ Sex: _____ Date of Birth: _____

Patient Identification Number: _____ Physician: _____

Vaccine	Dose, Site and Route of Administration	Date Given	Manufacturer	Lot #	Name, Title & Address of Person Giving Vaccine	Date Next Dose Due
Tetanus, Diphtheria Toxoids, for Adult Use (Td)						
Pneumococcal						
Influenza						
Measles						
Mumps						
Rubella						
Polio — OPV						
Polio — IPV						
Hepatitis B						
Others						
_____						
_____						
_____						

This form may be duplicated for use in patient files.

Appendix 8

Personal Immunization Record

Name: _____ Sex: _____ Date of Birth: _____

Address: _____

Vaccine	Date Given Month/Year	Doctor or Clinic Phone Number	Date Next Dose Due
Tetanus, Diphtheria Toxoids, for Adult Use (Td)	_____	_____	_____
	_____	_____	_____
	_____	_____	_____
	_____	_____	_____
Pneumococcal	_____	_____	_____
Influenza	_____	_____	_____
	_____	_____	_____
	_____	_____	_____
	_____	_____	_____
	_____	_____	_____
	_____	_____	_____
	_____	_____	_____
	_____	_____	_____
Measles	_____	_____	_____
Mumps	_____	_____	_____
Rubella			
Polio — OPV	_____	_____	_____
Polio — IPV	_____	_____	_____
Hepatitis B	_____	_____	_____
	_____	_____	_____
	_____	_____	_____
Others			
_____	_____	_____	_____
_____	_____	_____	_____
_____	_____	_____	_____

This form may be duplicated for distribution.

APPENDIX 9

Reportable Events Following Vaccination*

Vaccine/Toxoid	Event	Interval from Vaccination
DTP, P, DTP/Poliovirus combined	A. Anaphylaxis or anaphylactic shock	24 hours
	B. Encephalopathy (or encephalitis)[†]	7 days
	C. Shock-collapse or hypotonic-hyporesponsive collapse[†]	7-days
	D. Residual seizure disorder[†]	(*See* Aids to Interpretation)[†]
	E. Any acute complication or sequela (including death) of above events	No limit
	F. Events in vaccinees described in manufacturer's package insert as contraindications to additional doses of vaccine[‡]	(*See* package insert)
Measles, Mumps, and Rubella; DT, Td, T toxoid	A. Anaphylaxis or anaphylactic shock	24 hours
	B. Encephalopathy (or encephalitis)[†]	15 days for measles, mumps, and rubella vaccines; 7 days for DT, Td, and T toxoids
	C. Residual seizure disorder[†]	(*See* Aids to Interpretation)[†]
	D. Any acute complication or sequela (including death) of above events	No limit
	E. Events in vaccinees described in manufacturer's package insert as contraindications to additional doses of vaccine[‡]	(*See* package insert)
Oral Poliovirus vaccine	A. Paralytic poliomyelitis	
	– in a nonimmunodeficient recipient	30 days
	– in an immunodeficient recipient	6 months
	– in a vaccine-associated community case	No limit
	B. Any acute complication or sequela (including death) of above events	No limit

| | C. | Events in vaccines described in manufacturer's package insert as contraindications to additional doses of vaccine[‡] | (*See* package insert) |

Inactivated Poliovirus vaccine	A.	Anaphylaxis or anaphylactic shock	24 hours
	B.	Any acute complication or sequela (including death) of above event	No limit
	C.	Events in vaccinees described in manufacturer's package insert as contraindications to additional doses of vaccine[‡]	(*See* package insert)

* Events listed are required by law to be reported to the U.S. Department of Health and Human Services; however, the Vaccine Adverse Event Reporting System (VAERS) will accept *all* reports of suspected adverse events after the administration of *any* vaccine.

† **Aids to Interpretation**

Shock-collapse or hypotonic-hyporesponsive collapse may be evidenced by signs or symptoms such as decrease in or loss of muscle tone, paralysis (partial or complete), hemiplegia, hemiparesis, loss of color or change of color to pale white or blue, unresponsiveness to environmental stimuli, depression of or loss of consciousness, prolonged sleeping with difficulty arousing, or cardiovascular or respiratory arrest.

Residual seizure disorder may be considered to have occurred if no other seizure or convulsion unaccompanied by fever or accompanied by a fever of <102 °F occurred before the first seizure or convulsion after the administration of the vaccine involved AND, if in the case of measles-, mumps-, or rubella-containing vaccines, the first seizure or convulsion occurred within 15 days after vaccination OR in the case of any other vaccine, the first seizure or convulsion occurred within 3 days after the vaccination, AND, if two or more seizures or convulsions unaccompanied by fever or accompanied by a fever of <102 °F occurred within 1 year after vaccination.

The terms seizure and convulsion include grand mal, petit mal, absence, myoclonic, tonic-clonic, and focal motor seizures and signs.

Encephalopathy refers to any significant acquired abnormality of, injury to, or impairment of brain function. Among the frequent manifestations of encephalopathy are focal and diffuse neurologic signs, increased intracranial pressure, or changes lasting ≥6 hours in level of consciousness, with or without convulsions. The neurologic signs and symptoms of encephalopathy may be temporary with complete recovery, or they may result in various degrees of permanent impairment. Signs and symptoms such as high-pitched and unusual screaming, persistent unconsolable crying, and bulging fontanel are compatible with an encephalopathy, but in and of themselves are not conclusive evidence of encephalopathy. Encephalopathy usually can be documented by slow-wave activity on an electroencephalogram.

‡ Refer to the CONTRAINDICATION section of the manufacturer's package insert for each vaccine.
Source: MMWR 1990;39:730–3.

Appendix 10

Reporting of Events Occurring after Vaccination

Who Reports:	Health care providers, manufacturers, vaccine recipients, and parents/guardians of vaccine recipients
What Products To Report	**Mandated:** DTP, P, Measles, Mumps, Rubella, DT, Td, T, OPV, IPV **Voluntary:** Cholera, JE, HiB, HBV, Influenza, Meningococcal, Pneumococcal, Yellow Fever
What Reactions To Report	Events listed in Appendix 9 including contraindicating reactions specified in manufacturer's package insert
How To Report	Complete form VAERS-1, with or without assistance from health care provider
Where To Report	VAERS* P.O. Box 1100 Rockville, MD 20849-1100
Where To Obtain Forms	800-822-7967

* VAERS (Vaccine Adverse Event Reporting System) will accept ALL reports of suspected adverse events after the administration of ANY vaccine. VAERS is intended to provide a single focus for such reports, replacing the Centers for Disease Control and Prevention's Monitoring System for Adverse Events Following Immunization (MSAEFI) and the Food and Drug Administration's Adverse Reaction Reporting System for publicly and privately purchased vaccines, respectively.

Source: Centers for Disease Control and Prevention.

Appendix 11.

Selected Bibliography

General

1. Siber GR, Werner BG, Halsey NA, et al. Interference of immune globulin with measles and rubella immunization. *J Pediatr.* 1993;122:204-11.
2. Centers for Disease Control and Prevention. Recommendations of the Immunization Practices Advisory Committee (ACIP): general recommendations on immunization. *MMWR.* 1994;43(RR-1):1-39.
3. U.S. Preventive Services Task Force. *Guide to Clinical Preventive Services: An Assessment of the Effectiveness of 169 Interventions.* Baltimore: Williams & Wilkins; 1989.
4. Centers for Disease Control. Immunization recommendations for health-care workers. Atlanta: U.S. Department of Health and Human Services, Public Health Service; 1989.
5. Centers for Disease Control. National Childhood Vaccine Injury Act: reporting requirements for permanent vaccination records and for reporting selected events after vaccination. *MMWR.* 1988;37:197-200.
6. Centers for Disease Control. Health Information for International Travel. Atlanta, Georgia: Department of Health and Human Services, Public Health Service; 1989. HHS publication (CDC) 89-8280.
7. Plotkin SA, Mortimer EA Jr eds. *Vaccines.* Philadelphia: W.B. Saunders; 1988.
8. Root RK, Warren KS, Griffiss JM, Sande MA, eds. *Immunization.* New York: Churchill Livingstone; 1989.
9. Murray DL. Vaccine-preventable diseases and medical personnel. *Arch Intern Med.* 1990;150:25-6.
10. Poland GA, Love KR, Hughes CE. Routine immunization of the HIV-positive asymptomatic patient: clinical reviews. *J Gen Intern Med.* 1990;5:147-52.
11. Lavi S, Zimmerman B, Koren G, Gold R. Administration of measles, mumps, and rubella virus vaccine (live) to egg-allergic children. *JAMA.* 1990;263:269-71.
12. Gable CB, Holzer SS, Engelhart L, Friedman RB, Smeltz F, Schroeder D, Baum K. Pneumococcal vaccine. *JAMA.* 1990;264:2910-8.
13. Jonsson B. Cost-benefit analysis of hepatitis B vaccination. *Postgrad Med J.* 1987;63:27-32.
14. Krahn MD, Detsky AS. Universal hepatitis B vaccination: the economics of prevention. *Can Med Assoc J.* 1992;146:19-21.
15. Riddiough MA, Sisk JE, Bell JC. Influenza vaccination: cost-effectiveness and public policy. *JAMA.* 1983;249:3189-95.
16. Sisk JE, Riegelman RK. Cost effectiveness of vaccination against pneumococcal pneumonia: an update. *Ann Intern Med.* 1986;104:79-86.
17. Schaffner W, ed. Immunization in adults I and II. *Infect Dis Clin North Am.* 1990;4:1-173,179-354.

18. Fedson DS. Prevention and Control of Nosocomial Infections. In: Wenzel RP; ed. *Prevention and Control of Nosocomial Infections.* Baltimore: Williams & Wilkins;1993.

Implementation Strategies

1. Barton MB, Schoenbaum SC. Improving influenza vaccination performance in an HMO setting: the use of computer-generated reminders and peer comparison feedback. *Am J Public Health.* 1990;80:534-6.

2. Buffington J, Bell KM, LaForce FM, et al. A target-based model for increasing influenza immunizations in private practice. *J Gen Intern Med.* 1991;6:204-9.

3. Fedson DS. Influenza and pneumococcal immunization strategies for physicians. *Chest.* 1987;91:436-43.

4. Nichol KL, Korn JE, Margolis KL, et al. Achieving the national health objective for influenza immunization: success of an institution-wide vaccination program. *Am J Med.* 1990;89:156-60.

5. Nichol KL. Improving influenza vaccination rates for high-risk inpatients. *Am J Med.* 1991;91:584-8.

6. Pachucki CT, Walsh-Pappas SA, Fuller GF, et al. Influenza A among hospital personnel and patients: implications for recognition, prevention, and control. *Arch Intern Med.* 1989;149:77-80.

7. Schoenbaum SC. Developing effective systems for delivery of vaccines. *Infect Dis Clin North Am.* 1990;4:199-209.

8. Setia U, Serventi I, Lorenz P. Factors affecting the use of influenza vaccine in the institutionalized elderly. *J Am Geriatr Soc.* 1985;33:856-8.

9. Williams WW, Hickson MA, Kane MA, et al. Immunization policies and vaccine coverage among adults: the risk for missed opportunities. *Ann Intern Med.* 1988;108:616-25.

10. Poland GA, Nichol KL. Medical schools and immunization policies: missed opportunities for disease prevention. *Ann Intern Med.* 1990;113:628-31.

11. Fedson DS. Clinical practice and public policy for influenza and pneumococcal vaccination of the elderly. *Clin Geriatr Med.* 1992;8:183-99.

Accidental or Unavoidable Exposures

Botulism

1. Release of botulism antitoxin (published erratum appears in *MMWR.* 1986;35:522). *MMWR.* 1986;35:490-1.

2. Morris JG. Current trends in therapy of botulism in the United States. In: Lewis GE Jr; ed. *Biomedical Aspects of Botulism.* New York: Academic Press;1981:317-26.

3. Tacket CO, Shandera WX, Mann JM, et al. Equine antitoxin and other factors that predict outcome in type A foodborne botulism. *Am J Med.* 1984;76:794.

4. Lewis GE Jr, Metzger JF. Studies on the prophylaxis and treatment of botulism. In: Eaker D, Wadstrom T; eds. *Natural Toxins.* New York: Pergamon Press;1980:601-6.

5. Hatheway CL, Snyder JD, Seals JE, et al. Antitoxin levels in botulism patients treated with trivalent equine botulism antitoxin to toxin types A, B, and E. *J Infect Dis.* 1984;150:407.

6. Black RE, Gunn RA. Hypersensitivity reactions associated with botulinal antitoxin. *Am J Med.* 1980;69:567.

7. Wainwright RB, Heyward WL, Middaugh JP, et al. Food-borne botulism in Alaska, 1947-1985: epidemiology and clinical findings. *J Infect Dis.* 1988;157:1158.

Snake Bite

8. Gold BS, Barish RA. Venomous snakebites. Current concepts in diagnosis, treatment and management. *Emerg Med Clin North Am.* 1992;10:249-67.

9. Sprenger TR, Bailey WJ. Snakebite treatment in the United States. *Intern J Dermatol.* 1986;25:479-84.

10. Successful venomous snakebite neutralization with massive antivenim infusion in a child [Letter]. *J Trauma.* 1985;25:464-5.

11. Lindsey D. Controversy in snake bite—time for a controlled appraisal [Editorial]. *J Trauma.* 1985;25:462-3.

12. Wingert WA, Chan L. Rattlesnake bites in southern California and rationale for recommended treatment. *West J Med.* 1988;148:37-44.

Hepatitis C

13. Dolan PJ, Skibba RM, Hagan RC, Kilgore WR 3d. Hepatitis C: prevention and treatment. *Am Fam Physician.* 1991;43:1347-50.

14. Go GW, Baraff LJ, Schriger DL. Management guidelines for health care workers exposed to blood and body fluids. *Ann Emerg Med.* 1991;20:11341-50.

15. Gerberding JL, Henderson DK. Management of occupational exposures to blood-borne pathogens: hepatitis B virus, hepatitis C virus, and human immunodeficiency virus. *Clin Infect Dis.* 1992;14:1179-85.

16. Dienstag JL. Non-A, non-B hepatitis. II. Experimental transmission, putative virus agents and markers, and prevention. *Gastroenterology.* 1983;85:743-68.

17. Dindzans VJ. Viral hepatitis. Preexposure and postexposure prophylaxis. *Postgrad Med.* 1992;92:43-6,49-52.

Immunocompromised Adults

1. Rubin RH, Young LS; eds. *Clinical Approach to the Compromised Host.* 2nd ed. New York: Medical Book Company; 1988.

2. Linnemann CC Jr, First MR, Schiffman G. Revaccination of renal transplant and hemodialysis recipients with pneumococcal vaccine. *Arch Intern Med.* 1986;146:1554-6.

3. Collier AC, Corey L, Murphy VL, Handsfield HH. Antibody to human immunodeficiency virus and suboptimal response to hepatitis B vaccination. *Ann Intern Med.* 1988;109:101-5.

4. Siber GR, Weitzman SA, Aisenberg AC. Antibody response of patients with Hodgkin's disease to protein and polysaccharide antigens. *Rev Infect Dis.* 1981;3(Suppl):S144-59.

5. Rimola A, Soto R, Bory F, Arroyo V, Piera C, Rodes J. Reticuloendothial system phagocytic activity in cirrhosis and its relation to bacterial infection and prognosis. *Hepatology.* 1984;4:53-8.

6. Gross PA, Gould AL, Brown AE. Effect of cancer chemotherapy on the immune response to influenza virus vaccine: review of published studies. *Rev Infect Dis.* 1985;7:613-8.

7. Nelson KE, Clements ML, Miotti P, Cohn S, Polk BF. The influence of human immunodeficiency virus (HIV) infection on antibody responses to influenza vaccines. *Ann Intern Med.* 1988;109:383-8.

8. Onorato IM, Markowitz LE. Immunizations, vaccine-preventable diseases, and HIV infection. In: Wormser GP; ed. AIDS and other manifestations of HIV infection. 2nd edition. New York: Raven Press; 1992.

9. LaMontagne JR. Immunizations programs and human immunodeficiency virus. *Rev Infect Dis.* 1989;II(3)S639-43.

10. Lederman MM, Schiffman G, Rodman HM. Pneumococcal immunization in adult diabetics. *Diabetes.* 1981;30:119-21.

11. Wright PF, Hatch MH, Kasselberg AG, et al. Vaccine-associated poliomyelitis in a child with sex-linked agammaglobulinemia. *J Pediatr.* 1977;91:408-12.

12. Quinn TC. Interactions of the human immunodeficiency virus and tuberculosis and the implications for BCG vaccination. *Rev Infect Dis.* 1989;11(Suppl 2):S379-84.

13. Kaplan L, Daum RS, Smaron M, McCarthy CA. Severe measles in immunocompromised patients. *JAMA.* 1992;267:1237-41.

14. Carpenter CB. Immunosuppression in organ transplantation. *N Engl J Med.* 1990;322:1224-26.

15. Styrt B. Infection associated with asplenia: risks, mechanisms, and prevention. *Am J Med.* 1990;88:5-33N-42N.

16. Centers for Disease Control and Prevention. Recommendations of the Advisory Committee on Immunization Practices (ACIP): Use of vaccines and immune globulins in persons with altered immunocompetence. *MMWR.* 1993;42(RR-5):1-18.

International Travel

1. Gardner P, ed. Health issues of international travelers. *Infect Dis Clin North Am* 1992;6:275-502.

2. Wolfe MS, ed. Travel medicine. *Med Clin North Am.* 1992;76:1261-1497.

3. Studemeister A. Travel medicine for the primary care physician. *West J Med.* 1991;154:418-22.

4. Hill DR, Pearson RD. Health advice for international travel. *Ann Intern Med.* 1988;108:839-52.

5. Ferenchick GS, Havlichek DH. Primary prevention and international travel: infections, immunizations and antimicrobial prophylaxis. *J Gen Intern Med.* 1989;4:247-58.

6. Johnson PC, Ericsson CD, Morgan DR, et al. Lack of emergence of resistant fecal flora during successful prophylaxis of traveler's diarrhea with norfloxacin. *Antimicrob Agents Chemotherapy.* 1986;30:671-4.

7. Taylor DN, Sanchez JL, Candler W, et al. Treatment of traveler's diarrhea: ciprofloxacin plus loperamide compared with ciprofloxacin alone. *Ann Intern Med.* 1991;114:731-4.

8. Pitzinger B, Steffen R, Tschopp A. Incidence and clinical features of traveler's diarrhea in infants and children. *Pediatr Infect Dis J.* 1991;10:719-23.

9. Schultz M. Malaria in migrants and travelers. *Trans R Soc Trop Med Hyg.* 1989;83(Suppl):31-4.

10. Lobel HO, et al. Long-term malaria prophylaxis with weekly mefloquine. *Lancet.* 1993;341:848-51.

11. Centers for Disease Control. Revised dosing regimen for malaria prophylaxis with mefloquine. *MMWR.* 1990;39:630.

12. Winters RA, Murray HW. Malaria—the mime revisited: fifteen more years of experience at a New York City teaching hospital. *Am J Med.* 1992;93:243-6.

Hepatitis B

1. Centers for Disease Control. Hepatitis B virus: a comprehensive strategy for eliminating transmission in the United States through universal childhood vaccination: recommendations of the Immunization Practices Advisory Committee (ACIP).*MMWR.* 1991;40(RR-13):1-25.
2. McQuillan GM, Townsend TR, Fields HA, et al. Seroepidemiology of hepatitis B virus infection in the United States 1976 to 1980. *Am J Med.* 1989;87(Suppl 3A):5S-10S.
3. Alter MJ, Hadler SC, Margolis HS, et al. The changing epidemiology of hepatitis B in the United States. Need for alternative vaccination strategies. *JAMA.* 1990;263:1218-22.
4. Centers for Disease Control. Prevention of perinatal transmission of hepatitis B virus: prenatal screening of all pregnant women for hepatitis B surface antigen. *MMWR.* 1988;37:341-6, 351.
5. Mulley AG, Silverstein MD, Dienstag JL. Indications for the use of hepatitis B vaccine, based on cost-effectiveness analysis. *N Engl J Med.* 1982;307:644-52.
6. West DJ, Margolis HS. Prevention of hepatitis B virus infection in the United States: a pediatric perspective. *Pediatr Infect Dis J.* 1992;11:866-74.
7. Hall CB, Halsey NA. Control of hepatitis B: to be or not to be? *Pediatrics.* 1992;90:274-7.
8. Wainwright RB, McMahon BJ, Bulkow LR, et al. Duration of immunogenicity and efficacy of hepatitis B vaccine in a Yupik Eskimo population. *JAMA.* 1989;261:2362-6.
9. Krahn MD, Detsky AS. Universal hepatitis B vaccination: the economics of prevention. *Can Med Assoc J.* 1992;146:19-21.
10. Beasley RP, Hwang LY, Lin CC, et al. Hepatocellular carcinoma and hepatitis B virus. A prospective study of 22,707 men in Taiwan. *Lancet.* 1981;2:1129-33.
11. Centers for Disease Control. Intradermal administration of hepatitis B vaccine: an update. *Hepatitis Surveillance Report No. 54.* Atlanta: Centers for Disease Control, 1992; 2-5.
12. Hadler SC. Are booster doses of hepatitis B vaccine necessary? *Ann Intern Med.* 1988;108:457-8.
13. Hadler SC, Margolis HS. Hepatitis B immunization: vaccine types, efficacy, and indications for immunization. In: Remington JS, Swartz MN; eds. *Current Clinical Topics in Infectious Diseases.* Boston: Blackwell Scientific Publications;1992:282-308.

Immune Globulin

1. Dwyer JM. Intravenous therapy with gamma globulin. *Adv Intern Med.* 1987;31:111-35
2. Lassiter HA. Intravenous immunoglobulin in the prevention and treatment of neonatal bacteria sepsis. *Adv Pediatr.* 1992;39:71-99.
3. Sultan Y, Kazatchkine MD, Nydegger U, Rossi F, Dietrich G, Algiman M. Intravenous immunoglobulin in the treatment of spontaneously acquired factor VIII:C inhibitors. *Am J Med.* 1991;91:35S-39S.

4. Greenbaum BH. Differences in immunoglobulin preparations for intravenous use: a comparison of six products. *Am J Pediatr Hematol Oncol.* 1990;12:490-6.
5. Steele RW, Burks AW Jr, Williams LW. Intravenous immunoglobulin: new clinical applications. *Ann Allergy.* 1988;60:89-94.
6. Berkman SA, Lee ML, Gale RP. Clinical uses of intravenous immunoglobulins (published erratum appears in *Ann Intern Med.* 1990;112:967). *Ann Intern Med.* 1990;112:278-92.
7. Stiehm ER, Ashida E, Kim KS, Winston DJ, Haas A, Gale RP. Intravenous immunoglobulins as therapeutic agents (clinical conference) (published erratum appears in *Ann Intern Med* 1987;107:946). *Ann Intern Med.* 1987;107:367-82.
8. Pennington JE. Newer uses of intravenous immunoglobulins as anti-infective agents. *Antimicrob Agents Chemother.* 1990;34:1463-6.
9. Ballow M. Mechanisms of action of intravenous immunoglobulin therapy and potential use in autoimmune connective tissue diseases. *Cancer.* 1991;68:1430-6.
10. Ruiz de Souza V, Kaveri SV, Kazatchkine MD. Intravenous immunoglobulin (IVIg) in the treatment of autoimmune and inflammatory diseases. *Clin Exp Rheumatol.* 1993;11:S33-6.
11. Rosen FS. Putative mechanism of the effect of intravenous gamma-globulin. *Clin Immunol Immunopathol.* 1993;67:541-3.
12. Levinson AI. The use of IVIG in neurological disease. *Clin Rev Allergy.* 1992; 10:119-34.
13. Schwartz SA. Clinical use of immune serum globulin as replacement therapy in patients with primary immunodeficiency syndromes. *Clin Rev Allergy.* 1992; 10:1-12.
14. Siber GR, Snydman DR. Use of immune globulins in the prevention and treatment of infections. *Curr Clin Top Infect Dis.* 1992;12:208-56.
15. Stiehm ER. Recent progress in the use of intravenous immunoglobulin. *Curr Probl Pediatr.* 1992;22:335-48.
16. Pirofsky B, Kinzey DM. Intravenous immune globulins. A review of their uses in selected immunodeficiency and autoimmune diseases. *Drugs.* 1992;43:6-14.
17. Schwartz SA. Intravenous immunoglobulin (IVIG) for the therapy of autoimmune disorders. *J Clin Immunol.* 1990;10:81-9.
18. Cohen J. Intravenous immunoglobulin (IVIG) for gram-negative infection—a critical review. *J Hosp Infect.* 1988;12:47-54.
19. Recommendations of the Advisory Committee on Immunizaton Practices (ACIP): use of vaccines and immune globulins for persons with altered immunocompetence. *MMWR.* 1993;42:1-18.
20. Keller T, McGrath K, Newland A, Gatenby P, Cobcroft R, Gibson J. Indications for use of intravenous immunoglobulin. Recommendations of the Australasian Society of Blood Transfusion consensus symposium. *Med J Aust.* 1993;159:204-6.
21. Buckley RH, Schiff RI. The use of intravenous immune globulin in immunodeficiency diseases. *N Engl J Med.* 1991;325:110-1.
22. Shulman ST. Recommendations for intravenous immunoglobulin therapy of Kawasaki disease. *Pediatr Infect Dis J.* 1992;11:985-6.
23. Zanetti G, Glauser MP, Baumgartner J. Use of immunoglobulins in prevention and treatment of infection in critically ill patients: review and critique. *Rev Infect Dis.* 1991;13:985-92.

24. Nydegger UE. Intravenous immunoglobulin in combination with other prophylactic and therapeutic measures. *Transfusion.* 1992;32:72-82.

25. Ronda N, Hurez V, Kazatchkine MD. Intravenous immunoglobulin therapy of autoimmune and systemic inflammatory diseases. *Vox Sang.* 1993;64:65-72.

Influenza

1. Mast EE, Harmon MW, Gravenstein S, et al. Emergence and possible transmission of amantadine-resistant viruses during nursing home outbreaks of influenza A (H3N2). *Am J Epidemiol.* 1991;134:988-97.

2. Keitel WA, Cate TR, Couch RB. Efficacy of sequential annual vaccination with inactivated influenza virus vaccine. *Am J Epidemiol.* 1988;127:353-64.

3. Patriarca PA, Weber JA, Parker RA, et al. Risk factors for outbreaks of influenza in nursing homes. A case-control study. *Am J Epidemiol.* 1986;124:114-9.

4. Treanor JJ, Mattison HR, Dumyati G, et al. Protective efficacy of combined live intranasal and inactivated influenza A virus vaccines in the elderly. *Ann Intern Med.* 1992;117:625-33.

5. Arden NH, Patriarca PA, Fasano MB, et al. The roles of vaccination and amantadine prophylaxis in controlling an outbreak of influenza A (H3N2) in a nursing home. *Arch Intern Med.* 1988;148:865-8.

6. Gross PA, Quinnan GV, Rodstein M, et al. Association of influenza immunization with reduction in mortality in an elderly population: a prospective study. *Arch Intern Med.* 1988;148:562-5.

7. Ershler WB. Influenza vaccination in the elderly: can efficacy be enhanced? *Geriatics.* 1988;43:79-83.

8. Meiklejohn G, Hoffman R, Graves P. Effectiveness of influenza vaccine when given during an outbreak of influenza A/H3N2 in a nursing home. *J Am Geriatr Soc.* 1989;37;407-10.

9. Couch RB, Kasel JA, Glezen WP, et al. Influenza: its control in persons and populations. *J Infect Dis.* 1986;153:431-40.

10. Centers for Diseases Control and Prevention. Control of influenza A outbreaks in nursing homes: amantadine as adjunct to vaccine—1989-1990. *JAMA.* 1992;267:344-6.

11. Patriarca PA, Weber JA, Parker RA, et al. Efficacy of influenza vaccine in nursing homes. Reduction in illness and complications during an influenza A (H3N2) epidemic. *JAMA.* 1985;253:1136-9.

12. Schoenbaum SC. Economic impact of influenza. The individual's perspective. *Am J Med.* 1987;82:26-30.

13. Fedson DS. Clinical practice and public policy for influenza and pneumococcal vaccination of the elderly. *Clin Geriatr Med.* 1992;8:183-99.

14. Foster DA, Talsma AN, Furomoto-Dawson A, et al. Influenza vaccine effectiveness in preventing hospitalization for pneumonia in the elderly. *Am J Epidemiol.* 1992;136:296-307.

15. Centers for Diseases Control and Prevention. Prevention and control of influenza. Part 1. Vaccines. Recommendations of the Advisory Committee on Inmunization Practices. *MMWR.* 1993;42:1-14.

16. Centers for Disease Control and Prevention. Final results: Medicare influenza vaccine demonstration-selected states, 1988-92. *MMWR,* 1993;42:601-4.

17. Fedson DS, Wajda A, Nicol JP, et al. Clinical effectiveness of influenza vaccination in Manitoba. *JAMA.* 1993;270:1956-61.

Japanese Encephalitis

1. Rosen L. The natural history of Japanese encephalitis virus. *Ann Rev Microbiol* 1986;40:395-414.
2. Hoke CH, Nisalak A, Sangawhipa N, et al. Protection against Japanese encephalitis by inactivated vaccines. *N Engl J Med.* 1988;319:609-14.
3. Sanchez JL, Hoke CH, McCowan J, et al. Further experience with Japanese encephalitis vaccine. *Lancet.* 1990;335:972-3.
4. Tsai TF. Japanese encephalitis vaccines. In: Plotkin SA and Mortimer E; eds. *Vaccines.* 2nd edition. Philadelphia: W.B. Saunders (In press).

Measles

1. Krugman S. Further-attenuated measles vaccine: characteristics and use. Rev Infect Dis. 1983;5:477-81.
2. Markowitz LE, Preblud SR, Orenstein WA, et al. Patterns of transmission in measles outbreaks in the United States,1985-86. *N Engl J Med.* 1989;320:75-81.
3. Markowitz LE, Tomassi A, Hawkins CE, Preblud SR, Orenstein WA, Hinman AR. International measles importations United States, 1980-1985. *Intern J Epidemiol.* 1988;17:187-92.
4. Gustafson TL, Lievens AW, Brunell PA, Moellenberg RG, Buttery CM. Sehulster LM. Measles outbreak in a fully immunized secondary-school population. *N Engl J Med.* 1987;316:771-4.
5. Nkowane BM, Bart SW, Orenstein WA, Baltier M. Measles outbreak in a vaccinated school population: epidemiology, chains of transmission and the role of vaccine failures. *Am J Public Health.* 1987;77:434-8.
6. Mathias RG, Meekison WG, Arcand TA, Schechter MT. The role of secondary vaccine failures in measles outbreaks. *Am J Public Health.* 1989;79:475-8.
7. Krasinski K, Borkowsky W. Measles and measles immunity in children infected with human immunodeficiency virus. *JAMA.*1989;261:2512-6.
8. McLaughlin P, Thomas PA, Onorato I, et al. Use of live virus vaccine in HIV-infected children; a retrospective study. *Pediatrics.* 1988;82:229-33.
9. Atkinson WL, Orenstein WA, Krugman S. The resurgence of measles in the United States, 1989-1991. *Annu Rev Med.* 1992;43:451-63.
10. Hill DR, Pearson RD. Measles prophylaxis for international travel. *Ann Intern Med.* 1989;111:699-700.
11. Atkinson WL, Markowitz LE, Adams NC, Seastrom GR. Transmission of measles in medical settings—United States, 1985-1989. *Am J Med.* 1991;91(Suppl3B): 320-4S.
12. Sellick JA, Longbine D, Schifeling R, Mylotte JM. Screening hospital employees for measles immunity is more cost effective than blind immunization. *Ann Intern Med.* 1982;116:982-984.
13. Adcock LM, Bissey JD, Feighn RD. A new look at measles. *Pediatr Infect.* 1992;6: 133-148.
14. Kaplan LF, Daum RS, Smaron M, McCarthy CA. Severe measles in immunocompromised patients. *JAMA.* 1992;267:1237-41.

15. Committee on Infectious Diseases, American Academy of Pediatrics. *Report of the Committee on Infectious Diseases (Red Book)*. 22nd edn. Elk Grove Village, Ill: American Academy of Pediatrics; 1991:308-23.
16. Poland GA, Nichol KL. Medical students as sources of rubella and measles outbreaks. *Arch Intern Med*. 1990;150:44-6.
17. Raad II, Sherertz RJ, Rains CS, et al. The importance of nosocomial transmission of measles in the propagation of a community outbreak. *Infect Control Hosp Epidemiol*. 1989;10:161-6.
18. Markowitz LE, Preblud SR, Fine PE, Orenstein WA. Duration of live measles vaccine-induced immunity. *Pediatr Infect Dis J*. 1990;9:101-10.
19. Braunstein H, Thomas S. Immunity to measles in a large population of varying age. *Am J Dis Child*. 1990;144:296-298.
20. Lavi S, Zimmerman B, Koren G, Gold R. Administration of measles, mumps, and rubella virus vaccine (live) to egg-allergic children. *JAMA*. 1990;263:269-71.

Meningococcal Infections

1. Pinner RW, Gellin BG, et al. Meningococcal disease in the United States—1986. *J Infect Dis*. 1991;164:368-74.
2. de Moraes JC, Perkins BA, et al. Protective efficacy of a serogroup B meningococcal vaccine in Sao Paulo, Brazil. *Lancet*. 1992;340:1074-8.
3. Jackson LA, Wenger JD. Laboratory-based surveillance for meningococcal disease in selected areas, United States 1989-1991. *MMWR*. 1993;42(SS-2):21-30.

Mumps

1. Weibel RE, Buynak EB, McClean AA, Roehm ER, Hilleman MR. Persistence of antibody in human subjects of 7 to 10 years following administration combined live attenuated measles, mumps, and rubella virus vaccines. *Proc Soc Exp Biol Med*. 1980;165:260-3.
2. Cochi SL, Preblud SR, Orenstein WA. Perspectives on the relative resurgence of mumps in the United States. *Am J Dis Child*. 1988;142:499-507.
3. Chaiken BP, Williams NM, Preblud SR, Parkin W, Altman R. The effect of a school entry law on mumps activity in a school district. *JAMA*. 1987;257:2455-8.
4. Sosin DM, Cochi SL, Gunn RA, Jennings CE, Preblud SR. The changing epidemiology of mumps and its impact on university campuses. *Pediatrics*. 1989;84:779-84.
5. Wharton M, Cochi SL, Hutcheson RH, Bistowish JM, Schaffner W. A large outbreak of mumps in the post-vaccine era. *J Infect Dis*. 1988;158:1253-60.
6. Kaplan KM, Marder DC, Cochi SL, Preblud SR. Mumps in the workplace: further evidence of the changing epidemiology of a childhood vaccine-preventable disease. *JAMA*. 1988;260:1434-8.
7. Hersh BS, Fine PE, Kent WK, et al. Mumps outbreak in a highly vaccinated population. *J Pediatr*. 1991;119:187-93.
8. Wharton M, Cochi SL, Hutcheson RH, Schaffner W. Mumps transmission in hospitals. *Arch Intern Med*. 1990;150:47-9.
9. Lavi S, Zimmerman B, Koren G, Gold R. Administration of measles, mumps, and rubella virus vaccine (live) to egg-allergic children. *JAMA*. 1990;263:269-71.

Plague

1. Stollerman GH. Bacterial vaccines and toxoids: reviews of safety and efficacy. *Adv Intern Med*. 1978;23:405-34.

2. Williams JE, Cavanaugh DC. Measuring the efficacy of vaccination in affording protection against plague. *Bull World Health Organization.* 1979;57:309-13.

3. Cavanaugh DC, Elisberg BL, Llewellyn CH, et al. Plague immunization. V. Indirect evidence for the efficacy of plague vaccine. *J Infect Dis.* 1974;129:S37-40.

4. Recommendation of the Immunization Practices Advisory Committee (ACIP). Plague vaccine. *MMWR.* 1982;31:301-4.

5. Benenson AS. Immunization and military medicine. *Rev Infect Dis.* 1984;6:1-12.

Pneumococcal Infections

1. Janoff EN, Breiman RF, Daley CL, Hopewell PC. Pneumococcal disease during HIV infection. *Ann Intern Med.* 1992;117:314-24.

2. Shapiro ED, Berg AT, Austrian R, et al. The protective efficacy of polyvalent pneumococcal polysaccharide vaccine. *N Engl J Med.* 1991;325:1453-60.

3. Musher DM, Groover JE, Rowland JM, et al. Antibody to capsular polysaccharides of *Streptococcus pneumoniae:* prevalence, persistence, and response to revaccination. Clin Infect Dis. 1993;17:66-73.

4. Bennett NM, Buffington J, LaForce FM. Pneumococcal bacteremia in Monroe County, New York. *Am J Public Health.* 1992;82:1513-6.

5. Austrian R, Gold J. Pneumococcal bacteremia with special reference to bacteremic pneumococcal pneumonia. *Ann Intern Med.* 1964;60:759-76.

6. Simberkoff MS, Cross AP, Al-Ibrahim M, et al. Efficacy of pneumococcal vaccine in high risk patients: results of a Veterans Administration Cooperative Study. *N Engl J Med.* 1986;315:1318-27.

7. Forrester HL, Jahnigen DW, LaForce FM. Inefficacy of pneumococcal vaccine in a high-risk population. *Am J Med.* 1987;83:425-30.

8. Sims RV, Steinmann WC, McConville JH, King LR, Zwick WC, Schwartz JS. The clinical effectiveness of pneumococcal vaccine in the elderly. *Ann Intern Med.* 1988;108:653-7.

9. Bolan G. Broome CV, Facklam RR, Plikaytis BD, Fraser DW, Schlech WF III. Pneumococcal vaccine efficacy in selected populations in the United States. *Ann Intern Med.* 1986;104:1-6.

10. Huang KL, Ruben FL, Rinaldo CR Jr, Kingsley L, Lytes DW, Ho M. Antibody responses after influenza and pneumococcal immunization in HIV-infected homosexual men. *JAMA.* 1987;257:2047-50.

Poliomyelitis

1. Kim-Farley RJ, Bart KJ, Schonberger LB, et al. Poliomyelitis in the USA: virtual elimination of the disease caused by wild virus. *Lancet.* 1984;2:1315-7.

2. Nkowane BM, Wassilak SGF, Orenstein WA, et al. Vaccine-associated paralytic poliomyelitis. United States: 1973 through 1984. *JAMA.* 1987;257:1335-40.

3. Robertson SE, Traverso HP, Drucker JA, et al. Clinical efficacy of a new, enhanced-potency, inactivated poliovirus vaccine. *Lancet.* 1988;1:897-9.

4. Hinman AR, Koplan JP, Orenstein WA, Brink EW, Nkowane BM. Live or inactivated poliomyelitis vaccine: an analysis of benefits and risks. *Am J Public Health.* 1988;78:291-5.

5. Hinman AR, Koplan JR, Orenstein WA, Brink EW. Decision analysis and polio immunization policy. *Am J Public Health.* 1988;78:301-3.

6. Hinman AR, Foege WH, de Quadros CA, Patriarca PA, Orenstein WA, Brink EW. The case for global eradication of poliomyelitis. *Bull World Health Organization.* 1987;65:835-40.
7. Wright PF, Kim-Farley RJ, de Quadros CA, et al. Strategies for the global eradication of poliomyelitis by the year 2000. *N Engl J Med.* 1991;325:1774-9.
8. de Quadros CA, Andrus JK, Olive J, et al. Eradication of poliomyelitis: progress in the Americas. *PIDJ.* 1991;10:222-9.

Rabies

1. Fishbein DB, Pacer RE, Holmes DF, Ley AB, Yager P, Tong TC. Rabies preexposure prophylaxis with human diploid cell rabies vaccine: a dose-response study. *J Infect Dis.* 1987;156:50-5.
2. Bernard KW, Mallonee J, Wright JC, et al. Preexposure immunization with intradermal human diploid cell rabies vaccine: risks and benefits of primary and booster vaccination. *JAMA.* 1987;257:1059-63.
3. Baer GM, Fishbein DB. Rabies post-exposure prophylaxis. *N Engl J Med.* 1987;316:1270-2.
4. Warrington RJ, Martens CJ, Rubin M, Rutherford WJ, Aoki FY. Immunologic studies in subjects with a serum sickness-like illness after immunization with human diploid cell rabies vaccine. *J Allergy Clin Immunol.* 1987;79:605-10.
5. Remington PL, Shope T, Andrews J. A recommended approach to the evaluation of human rabies exposure in an acute-care hospital. *JAMA.* 1985;254:67-9.
6. Helmick CG, Tauxe RV, Vernon AA. Is there a risk to contacts of patients with rabies? *Rev Infect Dis.* 1987;9:511-8.
7. Fishbein DB, Baer GM. Animal rabies: implications for diagnosis and human treatment. *Ann Intern Med.* 1989;109:935-7.
8. Centers for Disease Control. Human Rabies—Texas, Arkansas, and Georgia, 1991. *MMWR.* 1991;40:765-9.
9. Warrell DA, Warrell MJ. Human rabies and its prevention: an overview. *Rev Infect Dis.* 1988;10:S726-31.
10. Centers for Disease Control. Rabies prevention—United States, 1991: recommendations of the Immunization Practices Advisory Committee (ACIP). *MMWR.* 1991;40(RR-3):1-19.

Rubella

1. Greaves WL, Orenstein WA, Hinman AR, Nersesian WS. Clinical efficacy of rubella vaccine. *Pediatr Infect Dis.* 1983;2:284-6.
2. Chu SY, Bernier RH, Stewart JA, et al. Rubella antibody persistence after immunization: sixteen year follow-up in the Hawaiian Islands. *JAMA.* 1988;259:3133-6.
3. Munro ND, Sheppard S, Smithells RW, Holzel H, Jones G. Temporal relations between maternal rubella and congenital defects. *Lancet.* 1987;2:201-4.
4. Orenstein WA, Bart KJ, Hinman AR, et al. The opportunity and obligation to eliminate rubella from the United States. *JAMA.* 1984;251:1988-94.
5. Preblud SR. Some current issues relating to rubella vaccine. *JAMA.* 1985;254:253-6.
6. Goodman AK, Friedman SM, Beatrice ST, Bart SW. Rubella in the workplace: the need for employee immunization. *Am J Public Health.* 1987;77:725-6.

7. Robertson SE, Cochi SL, Bunn GA, Morse DL, Preblud SR. Preventing rubella: assessing missed opportunities for immunization. *Am J Public Health.* 1987; 77:1347-9.

8. Tingle AJ, Yang T, Allen M, Kettyls GD, Larke RPB, Schulzer M. Prospective immunological assessment of arthritis induced by rubella vaccine. *Infect Immunol.* 1983;40:22-8.

9. Tingle AJ, Allen M, Petty RE, Kettyls GD, Chantler JK. Arthritis. Comparative study of joint manifestations associated with natural rubella infection and RA 27/3 rubella immunization. *Ann Rheum Dis.* 1986;45:110-4.

10. Benjamin CM, Chew GC, Silman AJ. Joint and limb symptoms in children after immunisation with measles, mumps, and rubella vaccine. *BMJ.* 1992; 304:1075-8.

11. Chen RT, Moses JM, Markowitz LE, Orenstein WA. Adverse events following measles-mumps-rubella and measles vaccinations in college students. *Vaccine.* 1991;9:297-9.

12. Lee SH, Ewert DP, Frederick PD, Mascola L. Resurgence of congenital rubella syndrome in the 1990s. *JAMA.* 1992;267:2616-20.

13. Tingle AJ, Allen M, Petty RE, Kettyls GD, Chantler JK. Rubella associated arthritis. I. Comparative study of joint manifestations associated with natural rubella infection and RA 27/3 rubella immunization. *Ann Rheum Dis.* 1986;45:110-4.

14. Tingle AJ, Pot KH, Yong FP, Puterman ML, Hancock EJ. Kinetics of isotype-specific humoral immunity in rubella vaccine-associated arthropathy. *Clin Immunol and Immol.* 1989;53:S99-S106.

15. Howson CP, Fineberg HV. The ricochet of magic bullets: summary of the Institute of Medicine report, adverse effects of pertussis and rubella vaccines. *Pediatrics.* 1992;89:318-24.

16. Centers for Disease Control. Rubella prevention. Recommendations of the Immunization Practices Advisory Committee. *MMWR.* 1990;39:1-18.

Tetanus and Diphtheria

1. Ballestra DJ, Littenberg B. Should adult tetanus immunization be given as a single vaccination at age 65? A cost-effectiveness analysis. *J Gen Intern Med.* 1993,8:405-12.

2. Prevots R, Sutter RW, Strebel PM, Cochi SL, Hadler S. Tetanus surveillance—United States, 1989-1990. *MMWR.* 1992;41:ss1-ss9.

3. Weiss BP, Strassburg MA, Feeley JC. Tetanus and diphtheria immunity in an elderly population in Los Angeles. *Am J Public Health.* 1983;73:802-4.

4. Crossley K, Irvine P, Warren JB, Lee BK, Mead K. Tetanus and diphtheria immunity in urban Minnesota adults. *JAMA.* 1979;242:2298-3000.

5. Ruben FL, Nagel J, Fireman P. Antitoxin responses in the elderly to tetanus-diphtheria immunization. *Am J Epidemiol.* 1978;108:145-9.

6. Simonsen O, Badsberg JH, et al. The fall-off in serum concentration of tetanus antitoxin after primary and booster vacination. *Acta Pathol Microbiol Scand.* 1986; 94:77-82.

7. Christenson B, Bottiger M. Epidemiology and immunity to tetanus in Sweden. *Scand J Infect Dis.* 1987;19:429-35.

8. Centers for Disease Control. Summary of notifiable diseases, United States, 1991. *MMWR.* 1991;40:57.

9. Chen RT, Broome CV, Weinstein, RA, Weaver R, Tsai TF. Diphtheria in the United States, 1971-81. *Am J Public Health.* 1985;75:1393-7.110.

10. Laforce FM. Routine tetanus immunizations for adults: once is enough. *J Gen Intern Med.* 1993;8:459-60.

Tuberculosis

1. Page MI, Lunn JS. Experience with tuberculosis in a public teaching hospital. *Am J Med.* 1984;77:667-70.

2. Geiseler PJ, Nelson KE, Crispen RG. Tuberculosis in physicians: compliance with preventive measures. *Am Rev Respir Dis.* 1987;135:3-9.

3. Slutkin G. Management of tuberculosis in urban homeless indigents. *Public Health Rep.* 1986;101:481-85.

4. Snider DE Jr. Bacille Calmette-Guérin vaccinations and tuberculin skin tests. *JAMA.* 1985;253:3438-9.

5. Villarino MA, Geiter LJ, Simone PM. The multidrug-resistant tuberculosis challenge to public health efforts to control tuberculosis. *Public Health Rep.* 1992;107:616-25.

6. Pust RE. Tuberculosis in the 1990s: resurgence, regimens, and resources. *South Med J.* 1992;85:584-93.

7. Hopewell PC. Impact of human immunodeficience virus infection on the epidemiology clinical features, management, and control of tuberculosis. *Clin Infect Dis.* 1992;15:540-7.

8. Onorato IM, McCray E, Field Services Branch. Prevalence of human immunodeficiency virus infection among patients attending tuberculosis clinics in the United States. *J Infect Dis.* 1992;165:87-92.

9. Edlin BR, Tokars JI, Grieco MH, et al. An outbreak of multidrug-resistant tuberculosis among hospitalized patients with the acquired immunodeficiency syndrome. *N Engl J Med.* 1992;326:1514-21.

Typhoid

1. Ryan CA, Hargrett-Bean NT, Blake PA. Salmonella typhi infections in the United States, 1975-1984: increasing role of foreign travel. *Rev Infect Dis.* 1989;11:1-7.

2. Edwards EA, Johnson JP, Pierce WE, Peckinpaugh RO. Reactions and serologic response to monovalent acetone-inactivated typhoid vaccine and heat-killed TAB vaccine when given by jet-injection. *Bull World Health Organization.* 1974;51:501-5.

3. Ferreccio C, Levine MM, Rodriguez H, et al. Comparative efficacy of two, three, or four doses of Ty21a live oral typhoid vaccine in enteric-coated capsules: a field trial in an endemic area. *J Infect Dis.* 1989;159:766-9.

4. Levine MM, Ferreccio C, Black RE, et al. Progress in vaccine against typhoid fever. *Rev Infect Dis.* 1989;11:S552-67.

5. Woodruff BA, Pavia AT, Blake PA. A new look at typhoid vaccination: information for the practicing physician. *JAMA.* 1991;265:756-9.

6. Acharya IL, Lowe CU, Thapa R, et al. Prevention of typhoid fever in Nepal with the Vi capsular polysaccharide of *Salmonella typhi. N Engl J Med.* 1987;317:1101-4.

7. Cumberland NS, Roberts JS, Arnold WSG, Patel RK, Bowker CH. Typhoid Vi: a less reactogenic vaccine. *J Int Med Res.* 1992;20:247-53.

Varicella Zoster

1. Gershon AA. Live attenuated varicella vaccine. *Annu Rev Med.* 1987;38:41-50.
2. Hayward A, Villanueba E, Cosyns M, Levin M. Varicella zoster virus (VZV)-specific cytotoxicity after immunization on nonimmune adults with Oka strain attenuated VZV vaccine. *J Infect Dis.* 1992;166:260-4.
3. Levin MJ, Murray M, Rotbart HA, Zerbe GO, White CJ, Hayward AR. Immune response of elderly individuals to a live attenuated varicella vaccine. *J Infect Dis.* 1992;166:253-9.
4. Gershon AA, LaRussa P, Hardy I, Steinberg S, Silverstein S. Varicella vaccine: the American experience. *J Infect Dis.* 1992;166:563-8.
5. Takahasi M, Ikatani T, Sasada K, et al. Immunization of the elderly and patients with collagen vascular diseases with live varicella vaccine and use of varicella skin antigen. *J Infect Dis.* 1992;166:558-62.
6. Berger R, Luescher D, Just M. Enhancement of varicella-zoster-specific immune responses in the elderly by boosting with varicella vaccine. *J Infect Dis.* 1984;149:647.
7. Gershon AA, Steinberg SP, LaRussa P, Ferrara A, Hammerschlag M, Gelb L. Immunization of healthy adults with live attenuated varicella vaccine. (published erratum appears in *J Infect Dis.* 1988;158:1149). *J Infect Dis.* 1988;158:132-7.
8. Gershon AA, Steinberg SP. Live attenuated varicella vaccine: protection in healthy adults compared with leukemic children. National Institute of Allergy and Infectious Diseases Varicella Vaccine Collaborative Study Group. *J Infect Dis.* 1990;161:661-6.
9. Gershon AA. Live attenuated varicella vaccine. *J Infect Dis.* 1985;152:859-62.
10. Ndumbe PM, Cradock-Watson JE, MacQueen S, et al. Immunization of nurses with a live varicella vaccine. *Lancet.* 1985;1:1144-7.
11. Hardy I, Gershon AA, Steinberg SP, LaRussa P. The incidence of zoster after immunization with live attenuated varicella vaccine. A study in children with leukemia. Varicella Vaccine Collaborative Study Group. *N Engl J Med.* 1991;325:1545-50.
12. Gershon AA. Varicella vaccine: still at the crossroads. *Pediatrics.* 1992;90:144-8.
13. White CJ, Kuter BJ, Hildebrand CS, et al. Varicella vaccine (VARIVAX) in healthy children and adolescents: results from clinical trials, 1987 to 1989. *Pediatrics.* 1991;87:604-10.
14. Asano Y, Nakayama H, Yazaki T, Kato R, Hirose S. Protection against varicella in family contacts by immediate inoculation with the live varicella vaccine. *Pediatrics.* 1977;59:3-7.
15. Watson BM, Piercy SA, Plotkin SA, Starr SE. Modified chikenpox in children immunized with the Oka/Merck varicella vaccine. *Pediatrics.* 1993;91:17-22.
16. Balfour HH Jr. Varicela zoster virus infections in the immunocompromised host. Natural history and treatment. *Scand J Infect Dis.* 1991;80(Suppl):69-74.

Yellow Fever

1. Centers for Disease Control. Yellow Fever. *MMWR.* 1990;39 (RR-10):1-5.
2. Woodall JP. Summary of a symposium on yellow fever. *J Infect Dis.* 1981; 144:87-91.
3. Poland JD, Calisher CH, Monath TP, Downs WG, Murphy K. Persistence of neutralizing antibody 30-35 years after immunization with 17D yellow fever vaccine. *Bull World Health Organization.* 1981;59:895-900.

4. Kaplan JE, Nelson DB, Schonberger LB, et al. The effect of immune globulin on the response to trivalent oral poliovirus and yellow fever vaccinations. *Bull World Health Organization.* 1984;62:585-90.

Future Trends

1. Lindberg AA, Norrby E, Wigzell, eds. Vaccines of the future: Nobel symposium 69. *Vaccine.* 1988;6:1-205.
2. The Jordan Report. A decade of progress. Accelerated development of vaccines. 1992. Division of Microbiology and Infectious Disseases, NIAID. Bethesda, Maryland: National Institutes of Health; 1992.
3. Bart KJ, Hinman AR, Jordan WS Jr. International symposium on vaccine development and utilization. *Rev Infect Dis.* 1989;11(Suppl 3):S491-667.
4. Centers for Disease Control. Progress toward achieving the national 1990 objectives for immunization. *MMWR.* 1988;37:613-7.
5. Morein B. The iscom antigen-presenting system. *Nature.*1988;332:287-8.
6. Parkman PD, Hopps HE. Viral vaccines and antivirals: current use and future prospects. *Annu Rev Public Health.*1988;9:203-21.
7. Halsey NA, Klein D. Maternal immunization. *Pediatr Infect Dis J.* 1990;9:574-81.
8. Sears SD, Clements ML, Betts RF, Massab HF, Murphy BR, Snyder MH. Comparison of live, attenuated H1N1 and H3N2 cold-adapted and avianhuman influenza A reassortant viruses and inactivated virus vaccine in adults. *J Infect Dis.* 1988;158:1209-19.
9. Baker CJ, Rench MA, Edwards MS, Carpenter RJ, Hays BM, Kasper DL. Immunization of pregnant women with a polysaccharide vaccine of group B streptococcus. *N Engl J Med.* 1988;319:1180-5.
10. Edwards KM, Decker MD, Graham BS, et al. Adult immunization with acellular pertussis vaccine. *JAMA.* 1993;269:53-6.
11. Hardy I, Gershon AA, Steinberg SP, LaRussa P, et al. The incidence of zoster after immunization with live attenuated varicella vaccine: A study in children with leukemia. *N Engl J Med.* 1991;325:1545-50.
12. Hayward A, Villanueba E, Cosyns M, Levin M. Varicella-zoster virus (VZV)-specific cytotoxicity after immunization of nonimmune adults with Oka strain attenuated VZV vaccine. *J Infect Dis.* 1992;166:260-4.
13. Robbins JB, Schneerson R. Polysaccharide-protein conjugates: a new generation of vaccines. *J Infect Dis.* 1990;161:821-32.
14. Levine M, Taylor DN, Ferreccio C. Typhoid vaccines come of age. *Pediatr Infect Dis J.* 1989;8:374-81.
15. Holmgren J, Clemens J, Sack DA, Svennerholm AM. New cholera vaccines. *Vaccine.* 1989;7:94-6.
16. Green KY, Taniguchi K, Mackow ER, Kapikian AZ. Homotypic and heterotypic epitope-specific antibody responses in adult and infant rotavirus vaccinees: implications for vaccine development. *J Infect Dis.* 1990;161:667-79.
17. Werzberger A, Mensch B, Kuter B, et al. A controlled trial of a formalin-inactivated hepatitis A vaccine in healthy children. *N Engl J Med.* 1992;327:453-7.
18. Amador R, Moreno A, Murillo LA, et al. Safety and immunogenicity of the synthetic malaria vaccine SPf66 in a large field trial. *J Infect Dis.* 1992;166:139-44.
19. Bockoff CA. Progress in the development of a vaccine against Plasmodium falciparum malaria. *Clin Microbiology Newsletter.* 1990;12:57-60.

20. Higashi GI. Vaccines for parasitic diseases. *Annu Rev Public Health.* 1988;9:483-501.

21. Ellerbeck E, Clements ML. AIDS vaccines. Supplement to Mandell, Douglas, Bennett's *Principles and Practice of Infectious Diseases.* New York: Churchill Livingstone; 1990:3-15.

22. Specter S, Lancz G. Problems associated with the developoment of a safe and effective human immunodeficiency virus vaccine. *Clin Microbiol Newsletter.* 1992;14:137-40.

Index